Language of the Feet

D0388214

written by

Chris Stormer
SRN, SCM, HV, RT

illustrated by
Michele Shayne Davey

Hodder & Stoughton

**For all the tremendous souls
in my life, and worldwide
particularly John, Andrew and David**

Orders: please contact Bookpoint Ltd, 130 Milton Park, Abingdon, Oxon OX14 4SB.
Telephone: (44) 01235 827720, Fax (44) 01235 400454. Lines are open from 9.00 – 6.00,
Monday to Saturday, with a 24 hour message answering service.
You can also order through our website: www.hodderheadline.co.uk

British Library Cataloguing in Publication Data

Stormer, Chris
  Language of the Feet
  I. Title
  615.822

  ISBN 0-340-64345-5

First published 1995
Impression number   20   19   18   17   16   15   14
Year   2004

Hodder Headline's policy is to use papers that are natural, renewable and recyclable
products and made from wood grown in sustainable forests. The logging and
manufacturing processes are expected to conform to the environmental regulations of
the country of origin.

Typeset by Wearset, Boldon, Tyne and Wear.
Printed in Great Britain for Hodder & Stoughton Educational, a division of Hodder
Headline, 338 Euston Road, London NW1 3BH by Cox & Wyman Ltd, Reading, Berkshire.

CONTENTS

ACKNOWLEDGEMENTS

Hodder and Stoughton
have come up trumps again! Thanks
to all those
involved in getting this book
off the ground!

Michele,
the artist, is to be commended for
her outstanding talent
and tremendous patience.
Well done, Michele,
and thank you!

Meanwhile to my loving family, John, Andrew and David;
my parents, Dick and Daphne; brother, Clive;
friends, especially Jenny and Val;
secretary, Liz; maid, Veronica;
tutors, Bev, Janine, Tracey, Wendy (in Harare)
and Elaine (in the United States of America);
all the RASA students and therapists,
and guides, especially Running Water;
colleagues and the media;
all of whom supported and encouraged me throughout
and never complained or begrudged me
the time or space to
complete this work,
THANK YOU!
I love you all!

INTRODUCTION

All healing forces are within.
The body can, and does, renew itself?

This book sets out to explain, in simple everyday language, feetspeak, chirology, pedology, and pedalology (an understanding of dis-ease by means of divination from the feet), so that ease can be re-established throughout the whole being. Its simplicity means that it can be enjoyed by everyone.

Feet, often taken for granted, are perceived to be either an asset or a hindrance, depending on feelings about the self and the quality of life. Not only do they support mind, body and soul through life's exhilarating and demanding adventures, but they constantly alter in appearance and consequence, to reflect outwardly the subtle fluctuations of the elusive and mysterious subconscious and unconscious minds.

The ever-changing characteristics of feet provide valuable clues as to inner needs and reflect potential for personal development and ultimate fulfilment.

Feet are remarkable! With 26 small bones, 19 muscles and over 30 ligaments, they adapt naturally to life's ups and downs, easily meeting the challenges of life. The only thing that interferes with this state of harmony is the mind! Feet sympathetically tune into thoughts and respond accordingly.

The marks of life's experiences impress the soul and soles, and are reflected on feet long before being mirrored in the physical body. Understanding these reflections allows for early detection of dis-ease, and prevents inner turmoil before damage occurs on all levels. Ill-fitting shoes do not cause foot disorders and discomfort, although they certainly exacerbate the condition.

Feet physically pampered by sensible, well-fitting footwear may still feel vulnerable and require extra emotional protection in the form of hard skin, bunions and corns. On the other hand, feet squeezed into ill-fitting, fashionable shoes can be totally relaxed and blemish free.

Distortions of the feet outwardly display distortions and misconceptions of the mind. Conformity to conflicting ethnic, social and parental beliefs, as well as conditioning, evokes various emotions from passive submission to resentment, anger, confusion, frustration and despair. Feet demonstrate the harmful influence of social conditioning which gives misplaced, unreasonable value to outdated beliefs and principles that limit and inhibit mind, body and soul, as well as the feet, by terrorising the whole. Urges to break free from social constraints are outwitted and overpowered by lack of confidence, uncertainty and the fear of possible ostracism. Those who do conform resign themselves to their fate by becoming dogmatic and unreasonable, due to the resultant deep fear and insecurity. Others resent being forced to behave in an alien manner, feeling it to be a burden and a curse. Either way, the emotion is immediately portrayed in the feet.

Feet reveal how potentially destructive and restrictive thought patterns can be reversed advantageously through a change of mind. Reflexology, an ancient and natural form of healing, helps release old disturbances and relieves mind, body and soul of burdens that otherwise hinder development. Understanding the language of the feet expands the therapy to embrace all emotional aspects of dis-ease, keeping pace with the inner needs of modern man.

The recent universal shift in consciousness encourages total dissipation of reluctance and fear to face personal truths, making space for enthusiasm and energy to resolve life's outstanding issues.

This book aims to instil the reader with the confidence and courage to release potentially harmful thought patterns willingly and mould a more constructive and creative reality. After all life is for living! Although the contents may elicit a variety of emotions, from total disbelief and denial to wonderment and conviction, keep an open, non-judgemental mind until fully experiencing and practising all that is offered.

The temptation to dismiss parts of the book as nonsensical arises from a reluctance to acknowledge threatening emotions that have been suppressed, by conventional belief systems, into the dark recesses of the mind. These are purposely or subconsciously ignored to avoid evoking internal havoc and mind-threatening confusion.

A naturally healthy body has beautifully formed feet, free of callouses and blemishes. Balanced in their view of life, their inherent tendency is to be flexible so that they can confidently stride ahead with love and joy, adapting spontaneously and appropriately to every situation.

Reading the feet is easy! As nature's gift to humanity, it offers long-awaited solutions for an improved way of life.

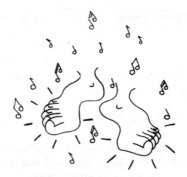

NATURALLY BALANCED FEET

THE PERFECT LIFE

The perfect life begins when there is no need for a better one!

What is the perfect life? After all, one person's stress is another individual's challenge!

- Life, if perceived to be an adventure, takes on totally new dimensions.
- Suddenly, stressful situations become challenging opportunities and fill the whole with vibrant energy and enthusiasm.
- Demanding experiences become exhilarating, testing previously unexploited inner characteristics that strengthen the soul.
- Life provides the choice – either to rise to each occasion and respond appropriately, or succumb and be defeated by the perceived pressures of social belief systems.

The language of the feet encourages the most beneficial choices to be made, by providing insight and knowledge for dramatic changes of attitude for self-improvement and an enhanced reality. The 'perfect' life can then begin!

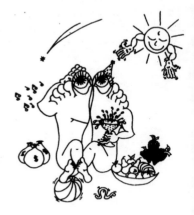

THE PERFECT LIFE?
ENJOYING THE PRESENT LIFE!

The only thing that is certain is that nothing is certain!

MIND POWER

The only thing that affects us is our own thinking!
A change of mind changes our life!

It is all in the mind – the brain minds the body and brings it to life!
The state of the body and feet are, therefore, outward reflections of
mindful activity. Negative ideas weigh down mind, body, soul – and
soles! The heavier the thought, the greater the burden and the more
swollen the feet.

Disharmony from mental confusion and emotional turmoil is
projected into the physical body causing dis-ease, pain and anxiety,
reflecting an unhappy state of mind. Thoughts of fear, hate and envy
create tension, havoc and confusion whilst loving thoughts relax
mind, body and soul, harmonising all bodily systems. It is easier than
imagined to replace uneasy thought patterns with healthy ones.

The language of the feet and Reflexology provide the option to
choose again and have a different experience! A change of mind lifts
individuals from limiting circumstances and places them on a journey
of self-discovery, with a life that contains all the elements of
happiness.

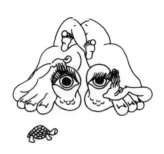

We only see the sunshine when we open the mind!

FEAT OF THE FEET

A firm foothold from which to grow and develop!

The incredibly designed feet support the massive bodily weight, even though only a relatively small area is in contact with the ground. Despite the thickness of the soles, an incredible amount of vibrancy is transferred from the ground, through the feet, to intermingle with ethereal energies absorbed into the body from the atmosphere. During health this absorption is powerful, forcefully reinforcing and strengthening the whole.

Mental tension and anxiety physically deprive the body of essential life-forces, making it increasingly vulnerable to disorders and disease. The soles are less supple and their resistance diminished, making them more impressionable.

The feet are considered our roots, metaphysically speaking. By turning our attention to them we can attain an inner peace and tranquillity. Deeper understanding of the meaning of life and gratitude for all that has preceded the present are essential steps in the healing process.

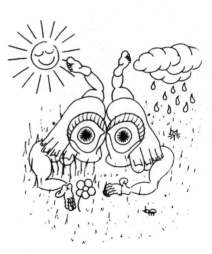

FEET – THE FIRM FOUNDATION FOR GROWTH AND DEVELOPMENT

Life is an adventure of the mind that makes the impossible possible!

READING THE FEET – A PRACTICAL GUIDE

A natural gift to mankind!

What are your feelings towards your feet? Have a good look! Note your initial impression:

- Do they please you?
- Are they ugly or embarrassing?
- Perhaps you feel attached to them?
- Is there any aspect you would like to alter or improve?

Feelings towards feet reflect the present subconscious perception of the self. As feelings change, so, too, do the characteristics of the feet. Feet tucked away in embarrassment indicate shyness and lack of confidence, whereas well-loved feet are displayed with pride.

Acceptance of the self allows for greater appreciation of the feet.

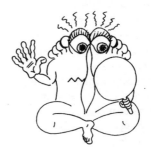

WHAT DO YOU THINK OF YOUR FEET?

Allow yourself to be yourself!
Don't worry about what others think – you may even
give them the courage to be themselves!
What a wonderful proposition!

USEFUL TIPS

*Through the Language of the Feet we shall learn
the truth and the truth will free us!*

- Reading feet is simple, but it is *emotive* for the recipient, so choose explanations with sensitivity, care and compassion.
- Never judge, condemn or criticise the self or others.
- Read feet with an open mind and trust the intuition. Relax! No effort is required!
- Position the recipient comfortably, with their bare feet raised to your eye-level.
- Sit directly opposite the feet.
- Use natural light for true impressions to be accurately interpreted.
- Look at feet whilst they are in a relaxed state, then ask the recipient to tense them, to determine bodily response to pressure.
- Prepare the recipient for the joyful relief of burdensome emotions that otherwise hinder development but which, temporarily, with recall, may evoke painful memories.

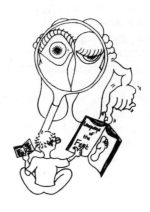

READING THE FEET. THERE IS MORE TO THE FEET THAN MEETS THE EYE

*Unlimited talents discovered through feet,
when unleashed, will benefit the whole of mankind.*

12 ✸

GENERAL OBSERVATIONS

Note your initial reaction on first seeing the feet. Then systematically observe the following:

- **General aspects** (page 14) for an overall impression of the whole.
- **Compare right and left feet** (page 17) to determine past and present impressions.
- **Relationship of the pair** (page 19) for interaction between the two.
- **Angle**s (page 20) to comprehend perimeters and direction.
- **Shape** (page 24) to ascertain personal characteristics.
- **Size** (page 28) to clarify dimensions.
- **Skin and nail** characteristics (page 29) to understand surfacing emotions that need to be released.
- **Temperature** (page 34) for the degree of emotion and its effect on the whole.
- **Colour** (page 33) to observe current moods. As moods do swing, colours change continually.

Reflexology footnotes

* FEET REFLECT PAST AND PRESENT PERCEPTIONS OF THE SUBCONSCIOUS MIND. THOUGHTS DETERMINE BODILY CONDITIONS AND MOULD FEET ACCORDING TO INHERENT AND ATTAINED BELIEF SYSTEMS.

* THE CONSCIOUS MIND'S TENDENCY INITIALLY TO REJECT MESSAGES FROM THE FEET ARISES FROM THE DISCOMFORT AND FEAR OF ACKNOWLEDGING SUPPRESSED EMOTIONS THAT CAN HURT.

* REFLEXOLOGY EFFECTIVELY RELAXES MIND, BODY AND SOUL, SO THAT OVERPOWERING EMOTIONS CAN BE RELEASED AND THE TRUTH ACKNOWLEDGED WITHOUT TRAUMA.

GENERAL ASPECTS OF THE FEET

Visualise bodily parts as reflected onto the feet in miniature. (Refer to the foot chart below.)

- The front of the body is mirrored onto the soles of the both feet, and the back of the body onto the tops of the feet.
- Energies of the right side of the body rebound onto the right foot, whilst energies of the left side of the body are reflected onto the left foot.
- Impressions and markings on the tops of feet reflect all that is perceived to be going on behind one's back.

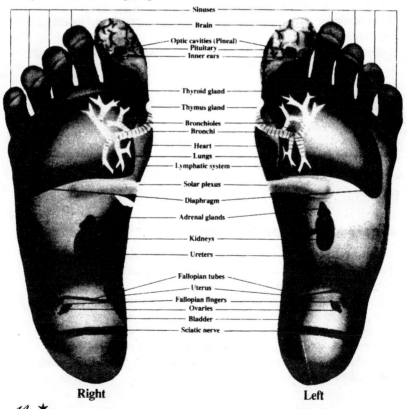

Sinuses
Brain
Optic cavities (Pineal)
Pituitary
Inner ears
Thyroid gland
Thymus gland
Bronchioles
Bronchi
Heart
Lungs
Lymphatic system
Solar plexus
Diaphragm
Adrenal glands
Kidneys
Ureters
Fallopian tubes
Uterus
Fallopian fingers
Ovaries
Bladder
Sciatic nerve

Right   Left

POSITION OF BODILY REFLEXES IN THE FEET

The toe pads: the head and face.

The toe necks: the neck and throat.

The hard ball: the bony ribcage, chest, breast and respiratory system and upper arms.

The fleshy instep: the soft abdominal region, the digestive system and parts of the reproductive and urinary systems.

The solid heel: the bony pelvis, lower reproductive system, lower urinary and digestive systems and lower limbs.

The top of the foot: the bony, muscular back.

The outer edge: the limbs, side of body and buttocks.

The inner edge: the spine and inner organs.

Each part reflects specific aspects of the subconscious and unconscious minds which ultimately determine the quality of life.

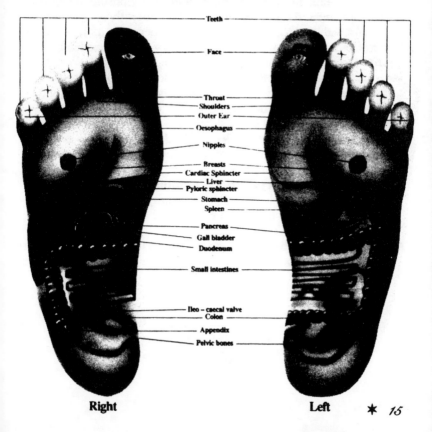

Teeth
Face
Throat
Shoulders
Outer Ear
Oesophagus
Nipples
Breasts
Cardiac Sphincter
Liver
Pyloric sphincter
Stomach
Spleen
Pancreas
Gall bladder
Duodenum
Small intestines
Ileo – caecal valve
Colon
Appendix
Pelvic bones

Right **Left** ✳ *15*

THE MEANING OF THE REFLEXES

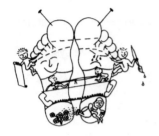

THE MEANING OF THE REFLEXES

Toes reflect thoughts. Like antennae, toes stretch into the universe to search for new thoughts and inspiration. Toe pads provide space to think and play around with ideas. By raising the level of consciousness, through stimulation of the toes, there is easier contact with the higher self and intuition becomes more acute.

Toe necks reflect expressions. They allow the free exchange of life's forces and the honest expression of the true self.

Balls of feet reflect feelings. They provide space for amicable feelings regarding the self and life in general by encouraging the full expansiveness of unconditional love through appropriate responses to each and every situation.

Upper half of the insteps reflect activities. They supply energy and enthusiasm to function constructively and effectively on all levels by being in control.

Lower half of the insteps reflect communications. They encourage pleasurable exchange of healthy communication and happy relationships by retaining beneficial aspects of life and discard detrimental ones.

Heels reflect mobility and security. The secure base from which to grow and develop, and the mobility to move ahead with ease and confidence.

*With the potential to become so much,
why settle for less?*

THE RIGHT (PAST) AND LEFT (PRESENT) FEET

Life is a journey, not a destination!

The characteristics of each foot provide substantial evidence that the right foot reflects past impressions, whilst the left foot is more impressed by the present. Both have a direct impact on the future.

Feet can be very different on the same person. A strict upbringing, for example, leaves no room for growth and development physically, emotionally or spiritually, stunting the growth of the right foot. Freedom from this inhibiting situation allows for expansion and growth and the left foot develops and grows accordingly.

- The outgoing and giving energies of the past (right foot) willingly impart their experience and wisdom to the present (left foot).
- The present (left foot) is receptive and openly receives advice and energies from the past (right foot) and energies in the present (left foot).
- Universal energy is moving from the masculine influence of the Piscean Age (right foot) into the female vibrancy of the present/future Aquarian Age (left foot).
- Light thrown on past (right foot) experiences, whether perceived good or bad, has a positive effect on life.
- The present/future (left foot) are filled with mystery and darkness and, therefore, vibrate to the negative tones, awaiting enlightenment and a raised level of consciousness through unconditional love and faith.
- The hollow vibrations of the right foot indicate past utilisation of supplies.
- The solidarity of the left foot provides substance and energy for present exploration and self-development.

Pythagoras was convinced that it was important to put the shoe on the right foot first!

- The liver reflex, mainly reflected on the right foot, stores memories and emotions of the past, whilst the spleen reflex on the left foot accumulates present emotions.
- With the bulk of the stomach reflex on the left foot, space is available for present experiences to be worked through. Anxiety and fear of future events creates stomach dis-comfort.

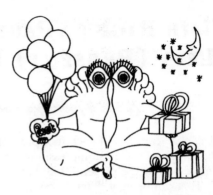

THE RIGHT AND LEFT FEET. THE FUTURE IS NOT WHAT IT USED TO BE!

(See Appendix II for summary.)

What lies behind and what lies ahead is insignificant to what lies in the present.

Reflexology footnote

* REFLEXOLOGY ENCOURAGES THE SUBCONSCIOUS MIND TO RELEASE TENSION ON ALL LEVELS, EASING THE WHOLE FROM THE GRIPS OF FEAR AND ANXIETY. AS IT DOES SO, THE FEET BECOME LIGHTER AND CHANGE THEIR OVERALL APPEARANCE.

THE SIGNIFICANCE OF THE PAIR

Be curious always for knowledge will not acquire us, we must acquire it!

Differences in the shape and size of a pair of feet provide valuable clues as to the influence of the past and present, as well as information regarding relationships. Look at the pair as a whole for an accurate interpretation.

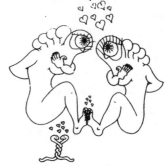

THE PAIR AND THEIR MEANINGS

Right foot masculine traits and relationships with men.

Left foot female characteristics and compatibility with females.

Tense right foot conflict with a particular male or several men, or resistance to the masculine aspects of the self or life.

Tense left foot dispute with female(s) or with the female principle.

General tension resistance to life in general and holding back.

Heavier right foot weighed down by unresolved emotions of the past.

Heavier left foot currently carrying a heavier load and more burdens.

Larger right foot less restricted in the past.

Larger left foot less inhibited in the present.

Smaller right foot restrained past.

Smaller left foot more confined in the present.

Misshapen right foot distorted by past pressures.

Misshapen left foot succumbing to pressures in the present.

Youth is not a time of life - it's a state of mind!

THE ANGLE OF THE FEET

Man is on a journey of self-discovery. The only limiting factor is himself?

Variations in the angle of the feet when walking or relaxed are noteworthy. The former indicates whether the approach is on track, whilst the latter demonstrates the immediate influence of the subconscious or unconscious minds.

Feet that hold back are reluctant to make an impression on the soul and soles. A spring in the step, or lack of it, demonstrates the quantity of enthusiasm and energy for life.

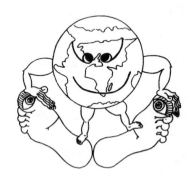

THE ANGLE OF THE FEET

POSITION WHEN WALKING OR STANDING

Natural feet: Parallel and point directly ahead.

Turned-in feet: Innate shyness, extreme self-consciousness or insecurity due to lack of confidence.

Turned-out feet: The degree to which feet point outwards indicates how far they are temporarily off track or imbalanced. Lack direction due to accommodating others, or following in the footsteps of others, or from taking orders or complying to instructions e.g. ballet dancers.

Tip-toe: Do not wish to create an impression or disturbance or draw attention to the self. Want to see more, raise status or attract attention.

Flat-footed: Totally dependent on others for support, e.g. babies and those with disabilities. Periods of being unsupported and discouraged.

Feet that step ahead with confidence are forthright in their approach and determined to get ahead. The weighty distribution of emotions and feelings throughout the whole determine foot and heel strikes e.g. a heavy outer heel strike indicates a reluctance and uncertainty about moving ahead due to inhibiting pressures within the family or society, arising from insecurity.

Continual shifts in thoughts and emotions alter inner tension, affecting the angle of the feet in the prone position. Refer to the chart below:

ANGLE OF THE FEET IN THE PRONE POSITION

	RIGHT PAST	LEFT PRESENT
Natural angle. Stand in an upright yet flexible position. Live for the here and now. Relaxed and balanced.		
Exhausted and weighed down. Significant past issues need to be acknowledged to prevent tendency to look ahead.		
Holding back something in the past but on track in the present.		
Being held back because living in the past. Need to let go to live in the present!		

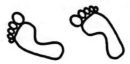

✱ *21*

Present progress temporarily inhibited because living in the past or looking back into the past for a solution to the present situation.

Addressing past issues in the present. Looking for solutions.

Wanting to move ahead. Living in the future.

Turning inwards for the answers or withdrawing from society to protect the self and exclude the outside world. Hiding true emotions. Avoiding exposure.

Soles turn in.

Drawing in to the self during periods of uncertainty, insecurity or depression. Lack of self-confidence. Introverted.

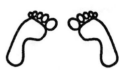

Turning away from having to confront inner feelings and emotions.

Soles turn away from each other.

A collapsed arch, in which the foot bows over the soles, needs to stand up for itself and not give into pressure. Inner substance required to believe in the self.

Collapsed arch.

RIGHT   **LEFT**
PAST   **PRESENT**

Prominent bunions draw the balls
of the feet together. Need to
liberate unresolved emotions to feel
less trapped.

A foot that appears shorter than the
other is either holding back or
fearful of being too obvious.
Self-confidence required.

       Shorter
       appearance.

A foot that looks longer, and possibly
more menacing, and putting 'its foot
down' is being more dominant and
very persistent! Seeking attention and
recognition.

       Longer
       appearance.

Reflexology footnote

✶ SOLES THAT TURN IN TO FACE ONE ANOTHER ARE PARTICULARLY COMMON ON
AUTISTIC AND DISABLED PEOPLE.

THE SHAPE OF THE FEET

Life's unique experiences entitle everyone to be an individual!

The overall shape of the foot reveals personal characteristics, aspects of upbringing, cultural beliefs and inherited attitudes, as well as the effect of past and current emotions.

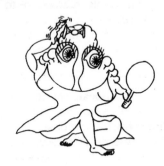

THE CHARACTERISTIC SHAPE OF THE FEET

CHARACTERISTICS AND SHAPE OF THE FEET

Flexible feet: Adapt easily and willingly to life's ups and downs. Versatile, supple and and complacent. If too flexible, easily manipulated.

Rigid feet: Harsh, strict, precise and highly principled. Need to believe in themselves more so that they feel less insecure, allowing for greater flexibility. Mental mobility will liberate the whole from unbending, unaccommodating ways.

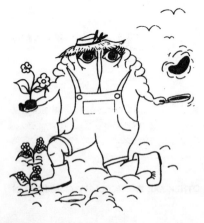

Broad feet: Support capable, down-to-earth people. Generally reliable and hard-working, organised and methodical, but rather impressionable. May have a tendency to 'put their foot in it'!

BROAD FEET: PRACTICAL AND DOWN-TO-EARTH

Narrow feet: A more aesthetic personality with a gentler and more sensitive nature. Enjoys being pampered and prefers others to do the menial tasks. Needs to expand to prevent confining and restricting themselves so that they have a broader approach to life!

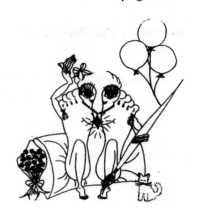

NARROW FEET: ENJOY AESTHETIC QUALITIES!

Straight feet: Uniform edges, with a straightforward approach to life, keeping to the straight and narrow e.g. track runners. Need to be cautious of being too direct and candid in their dealings and break away from their confined parameters to explore the unexpected.

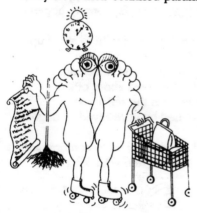

Functional feet: Large soles with inflexible, possibly insignificant toes, with little or no time for thoughts or imagination since the demands of the physical world take greater priority.

FUNCTIONAL FEET: CAUGHT UP IN THE PHYSICAL WORLD

Philosophical feet: Large big toes with distinctive pads on all toes. A good head, full of ideas and business acumen. Capable of vigorous, decisive activity and although they enjoy wisdom and moral philosophy, an active pastime would allow ideas to be put into practice!

Psychic/intuitive feet: Straight tops to some toes but all with long necks. They have their heads in the clouds and have little or no concern for the physical world. Belong to dreamers, and those with ethereal qualities, who are open to receiving universal knowledge. Need to keep their 'feet firmly on the ground'!

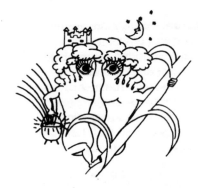

PSYCHIC/INTUITIVE FEET: WITH THEIR HEAD IN THE CLOUDS

Forlorn feet: Rejected, deprived or abandoned. Desperate and hopeless. Belief in the self will dissipate these emotions.

Light, unblemished feet: 'Foot-loose and fancy-free'. Happily adapt and go with the flow. Perceive only good in life. Forever hopeful and positive.

Floppy feet: Little or no inner substance and not able to stand up for the self. Needs to boost the self-esteem.

Ultra-sensitive feet: Impressionable, insecure and uncertain. If ticklish and dislikes being touched, concerned about others' opinions and feelings. Needs to believe in the self.

Heavy foot: Weighed down and burdened by unresolved or ongoing emotions that need to be released.

Squashed foot: Crushed, suppressed or constrained to conform and blend in with social and dogmatic belief systems. Lacking individuality and own ideas.

Mixed feet: Diverse qualities. For example: philosophical toes with short, practical necks and unusually elegant soles, that function mainly in the intellectual realm, but utilise their physical skills for pleasurable, creative amusements to rest the mind.

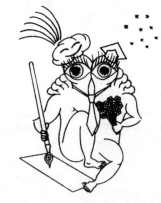

MIXED FEET: MULTI-TALENTED

Misshapen feet: Given in to relentless pressure and subconsciously cast to conform to inappropriate belief systems. Moulded to suit other belief systems resulting in feeling a misfit. Need to rediscover own identity.

Swollen feet: Unhappy, inhibited, disillusioned and drag their way through life. Weighed down with unresolved emotions. Unable to contain the self.

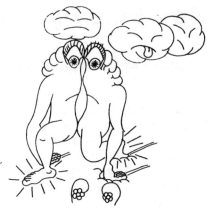

SWOLLEN FEET: WEIGHED DOWN WITH UNRESOLVED EMOTIONS

Disabled feet: Misdirected energy, misguided through mistaken belief systems and professional conditioning. The smooth skin allows impressions to slip away without lasting effects. Flat feet arise from the total dependence on others for support.

Abused feet: Attack of the self for not living up to expectations and belief systems. Do not feel worthy to deserve better.

Victimised feet: Perceive that they are not good enough. Invite abuse to reinforce this belief or to prove to themselves that they can survive despite the odds. Need to believe in themselves.

Autistic feet: Withdraw to escape life's harsh realities. Large toes with active minds, capable of tremendous imagination but the insignificant soles reflect the inability to put their ideas and thoughts into action.

Bound feet e.g. Chinese: Severe conformity to strict social belief systems, where personal impressions are not allowed, with no room for individual thoughts. Totally bound and subservient.

Reflexology footnotes

* THE REMARKABLY BLAND, UNBLEMISHED APPEARANCE OF FEET, PARTICULARLY AMONGST THE DISABLED, ABUSED AND AUTISTIC, MASKS TRUE EMOTIONS AND FORMS A PROTECTIVE OUTER SHELL.
* REFLEXOLOGY, WITH DOLPHIN MUSIC, LIBERATES THESE SPECIAL SOULS, GIVING THEM THE CONFIDENCE TO RELATE NATURALLY WITHIN THEIR SURROUNDINGS.

THE SIZE OF THE FEET

Laugh at yourself, and your feet, before others do!

Just as the body comes in various shapes and sizes, so it is with feet. Feet are not always in proportion with the body: some short people have large feet, and vice versa.

Some feet look as though they do not belong to the body to which they are attached! They are so out of character! This is because emotions have been so suppressed that a totally alien image is being projected.

Foot dimensions determine the type and degree of impression that a person is prepared to make or have made on them. Those with unnaturally small feet tend to limit themselves or do not feel that they need to make a great impression, whilst those with uncharacteristically large feet are more expansive in their approach to life.

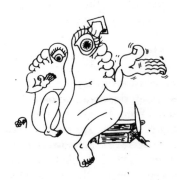

DIFFERENT SIZED FEET AND THEIR IMPRESSIONS

Large feet are capable of making a big impression if full potential is achieved.

Tiny feet tend to tread carefully to test their way through life, and although capable of making an impact, have a gentler approach.

Reflexology footnote

* SHOES DO NOT CAUSE FOOT DISORDERS BUT DO CREATE TEMPORARY IMPRESSIONS BY MARKING THE SKIN ON THE FEET. THE DEGREE DEPENDS ON THE AMOUNT OF INNER TENSION AND ANXIETY.

SKIN DEEP

Skin reflects camouflaged subconscious thoughts, feelings and emotions through its colour, texture and condition. Ticklish skin is exceptionally sensitive and requires careful handling since it indicates extreme self-consciousness.

Fluctuations in the nature of skin indicates mood shifts, influenced by feelings about the self, and present circumstances.

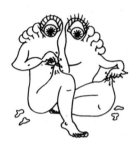

A CLOSER LOOK AT THE SKIN!

CHARACTERISTICS OF THE SKIN

Soft and pliable: Adapts spontaneously to life's experiences and responds appropriately to all situations.

Excessively soft: Lacks substance. Potentially lazy and hesitant. Enjoys voluptuous pleasure. Requires inner strength.

Flaccid: No energy, enthusiasm or strength. Gives in easily. No substance or definite direction. Needs to be more resolute.

Oedema: Overburdened and filled with unresolved burdens that prove weighty and inhibitive. Needs to unshackle the self of perceived burdens.

Hardened: Adamant, impenetrable, defensive, protective, impervious, stubborn. Concealing something. Hardened senses and firm ideas. Needs a more relaxed approach.

Sensitive: Vulnerable, self-conscious and impressionable. Easily hurt. Requires inner security.

Shiny: Emotional friction from rubbing up against perceived resistance or barriers. Worn away. Reflecting back emotions in the hope that others will be more understanding. Needs to feel secure and be less categorical.

Rough: Undergoing a strained, stormy, disorderly, harsh time. A level head and calm mind soothe the path of life!

Flaking: Extreme irritability at others or circumstances 'getting under the skin'. Needs a change and to be more tolerant of the self and others.

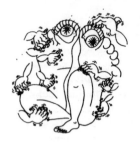

FLAKING, IRRITABLE SKIN. FED UP WITH LIFE GETTING UNDER THE SKIN

Athlete's foot: Ideas perceivably rejected causing great irritation and frustration. Requires acknowledgement and recognition.

Fragile: Delicate and easily hurt. Needs to boost self-esteem.

Smooth and dry: Exposed feelings and quick to take offence. A relaxed approach will ease the way.

Blistered: Friction and inner burning that has surfaced.

Blood blister: Internal hurt and grief from friction. Fill with compassion.

Wrinkled: Troubled and drained. Sapped of energy. Needs to stop worrying and being so concerned about the self and others!

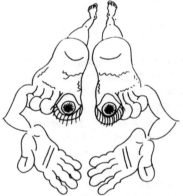

WRINKLED SKIN. ALWAYS CONCERNED AND WORRIED ABOUT OTHERS

Thick and hard: Thick skinned, impenetrable, insensitive, stubborn and extremely insecure, with a strong will and argumentative streak. Needs to be less dependent on the physical aspects of life.

'Extra' layer mask: Conceals true identity but should honestly express the self.

Rubbery feet, plastic appearance: Artificial and false, lacking zest or vitality. Unpenetrable and vulnerable, especially during periods of uncertainty and possible exposure.

Callouses: Emotional barriers that protect related areas of extreme vulnerability. Needs to go with the flow and believe in the self.

Flaking skin over callous: Irritable at having to conceal true thoughts, feelings and emotions. Friction from unresolved conflict. Needs to be more tolerant of the self and others.

Peeling: Extreme agitation. Allow the layers to peel away for a fresh start.

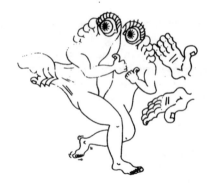

PEELING SKIN: SHEDDING THE OLD
TO MAKE WAY FOR THE NEW

Isolated hardness: Built-up resistance to certain issues or events, protecting the the self from exposure or hurt.

Cracked: Divided and torn apart. Separating two areas. Needs to trust the process of life.

Deep crevices: Feeling 'cut up' or divided. Go with the flow!

Blood capillaries: Inner emotional trauma and grief coming to the surface. Release with love and understanding.

Prominent, bulging capillaries: The emergence of subconscious hurts and unresolved issues that need to be released.

Silver lining or colouring: Universal help is at hand to guide and comfort.

White dots: Eruption of unexpressed emotions, particularly anger, frustration and jealousy. Let go!

Pronounced toe and foot print: An individual who likes to be identified with their own thoughts and actions.

Sores: Fresh hurts and open wounds.

Wounds: Old injuries leaving their mark.

Scars: Remnants of past pain, the memory of which is often concealed.

Warts: Unpleasant thoughts and concepts that are projected onto the surface. Look for the good!

Plantar warts: Extreme frustration at resources being tapped. Needs to be more resourceful!

Ulceration: Exposed deep fear that eats away at the self. Requires inner strength and a deep understanding of life's processes.

Dirt: Covers true vulnerability and self-consciousness. Hiding or feeling dirty. Wash the hands of wasteful emotions!

Pieces of grass, fluff and so on: Extra loads that are dispensable!

Temporary markings: From socks or shoes, display momentary impressions. e.g. the weave of a sock indicates the feeling of being caught up in a net or a line; a seam indicates a temporary division.

Itching: Irritable or a deep yearning e.g. itching to move on if in the heel, or itching to resolve issues if in the instep!

Swellings and lumps: Accumulated emotional congestion.

Reflexology footnotes

* CRAMPING IS OCCASIONALLY EXPERIENCED WHEN RECEIVING REFLEXOLOGY INDICATING:
    * A BELIEF THAT INDIVIDUALITY AND PERSONAL STYLE ARE BEING CRAMPED.
    * A GRIPPING FEAR OR EXTREME ANXIETY.
    * HOLDING TIGHTLY ONTO SOMETHING AND RELUCTANT TO LET GO.
    * EXTREME RESISTANCE.
* AS THE ENERGIES LEAVE THE BODY IN DEATH, ALL IMPRESSIONS OF THE PHYSICAL WORLD DISAPPEAR, LEAVING THE SKIN SMOOTH, COLOURLESS AND INDISTINCTIVE.
* ACHING, DURING OR AFTER REFLEXOLOGY, IS THE PHYSICAL MANIFESTATION OF SUBCONSCIOUS ANGUISH, DISTRESS, HURT, PAIN AND DISCOMFORT.

Colouring and Changing Moods of the Feet

As facial expressions change to reflect fluctuating moods, so too do the idiosyncrasies and coloration of feet. Overall shades echo predominant emotions, whilst contrasting tinges mirror varied emotions or inner turmoil. A patchwork display, with combined or overlapping tones, is common.

Colour variations as the feet relax, tense or stretch reveal the effect of deeply suppressed emotions under duress.

Colours of the Feet

Flesh coloured: Healthy, confident and balanced.

White: Drained of emotion or energy. Washed out. Exhausted. Trying too hard.

Red: Embarrassed, self-conscious, angry or frustrated. Need to feel at ease.

Yellow/orange: Totally fed up. Resentful, indignant and displeased. Jaundiced view of life.

Bluish/purple: Injured pride, bruised ego and battered self-esteem. Perceived emotional or physical abuse. Be kind to the self!

Green: Extreme envy, bitter, discontent and dissatisfied. Look for the good!

Brown: Browned off, bored or fed up!

Black marks: Deep emotional stabs. Perceived danger or difficulty. Need to trust the process of life!

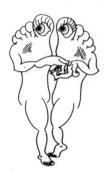

Embarrassed feet: Extremely self-conscious!

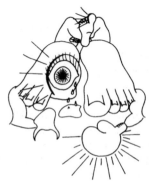

Angry, frustrated feet. Feeling out of control!

TEMPERATURE OF THE FEET

The vacillating degrees of bodily heat, emitted from the feet, demonstrate fluctuations in the intensity of feelings and emotions.

Warm feet: Glow with animated enthusiasm and temperate energy.

Burning feet: Inflamed and angry with a consuming need to express fuming emotions and move recklessly ahead.

Cold feet: Faint, weak, unexcited, unenthusiastic or disinterested. Initial confidence replaced by a reluctance to make the first move due to 'cold feet' at the last minute. Even cold weather can be demotivating!

A variety of emotions are unconsciously evoked and released during Reflexology. One foot may feel icy cold whilst the other is boiling hot. For example, the right foot may freeze at the subconscious arousal of past, unresolved emotions, whereas the left foot feels heated by the intensity of present emotions.

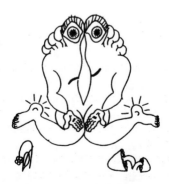

FLUCTUATING EMOTIONS

THE NAILS

Nails, the horny coverings on the outer tips of fingers and toes, protect the tips of the fingers and toes, especially from threatening outer forces. Toe nails reflect the cranial reflexes and protect, support and provide backing to thoughts, ideas and decisions.

TOE NAILS AND THEIR MEANINGS

Big toe: Defends personal ideas, intuition, thoughts and life's expressions.

Second toe: Cherishes concepts of the self and thoughts regarding feelings, emotions and unconditional love.

Third toe: Shields perceptions concerned with activity and control.

Fourth toe: Looks after thoughts regarding communication, relationships and pleasure.

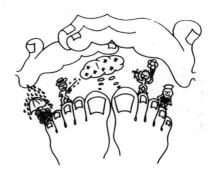

CHARACTERISTIC TOE NAILS

Little toe: Covers concepts of expansion, mobility and security influenced by perceptions of the family.

THE INFLUENCE OF THE SUBCONSCIOUS MIND ON THE NAILS

Ridged nails: Personal thoughts in opposition to other ways of thinking.

Horizontal: Weaknesses indicate periods of dis-ease and vulnerability.

Vertical: Fiercely protecting certain aspects of a particular perception.

Very ridged: Insecure due to perceived obstacles. Uncertain about protecting certain ideas.

Split nails: Divided and undecided about which thoughts to protect, those of the self or others. Wanting to break away from pleasing everyone.

Spoon-shaped: Depressed in the centre from lack of strength to defend personal decisions.

Hang nails: A strip of excess epidermis down the side reinforces or provides extra support to protecting perceptions and ideas.

Ingrown nail: The nail grows back into the skin from a deep need to protect ideas. Thoughts threatened and vulnerable.

Involuted nail – hollow underneath: Withdrawing from having to defend perceptions, yet gripping onto personal concepts despite uncertainty.

No nail: Unprotected. Feeling vulnerable and exposed. Lacking the substance or strength to back own thoughts and ideas.

Nail tearing: Continually pulling strips off the self, or perceiving others to be doing so. Removing protection to reveal vulnerability. Feeling exposed.

Broken nail: Wanting to break free from always having to be on the defensive.

Thickened nail: Feel that extra protection is necessary.

Weakness: Periods of debilitation, exhaustion and feebleness.

Bruised nail: Hurt at resistance met in protecting ideas. Unhappy about having to guard decisions.

Short nails: Like to keep in touch.

Fungal infection: Inflamed at feeling vulnerable and taken advantage of. The extra thickness provides added protection.

Yellow nail: Fed up at having to protect and justify thoughts and ideas.

THE KNOWLEDGE OF THE TOES

Man's mind, once stretched by knowledge and new ideas, never goes back to its original dimensions!

Toes reflect perceptions of the subconscious and unconscious minds, whilst soles reflect how these thoughts and ideas are put into action to create individual reality.

Toes, as individual balancers, reach out, like antennae, to seek universal knowledge and explore life to the full. Being 'on the toes', conveys an eagerness and enthusiasm for life, which can be enhanced through Reflexology, through the massage and stimulation of the

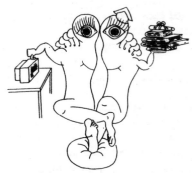

IT'S ALL IN THE TOES!

head, brain, face and sensory reflexes, on the toes. Thought patterns reflected onto the toe pads include those of:

The subconscious mind: the depth at which fears, anxieties and anger are suppressed and hidden in the recesses of the mind.
The unconscious mind: the plane of automatic functioning, such as breathing, for survival.
The conscious mind: the level of alert mental awareness.

Each toe symbolises a specific aspect of the mind, with significant consciousness being immediately mirrored onto the toe pads. For this reason the toes should be studied in their entirety as well as separately.

Knowledge replaces an empty mind with an open one!

TOE PERCEPTIONS

A wise man alters his life by altering his thinking!

Collectively and individually toes reflect the working of the mind and the biography of the soul!

Right toes reveal past thoughts and perceptions.
Left toes display present ideas and perceptions.
Length and shape portray individual potential.

TOE QUALITY

Flexible toes: Are secure, alert, yet relaxed and adapt well with mobility of thought. Others are encouraged to think for themselves. Too much flexibility encourages manipulation.

Rigid toes: Feel insecure. Lack mental flexibility and are easily irritated. Have very definite ideas and like others to conform to them.

The Big Toe/The Thinking Toe

Reflects intuitive, intellectual thoughts that expand beyond physical limitations into the expansive ethereal and spiritual realms.

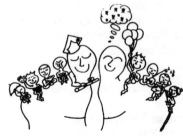

Second Toe/The Feeling Toe

Mirrors perceptions of the self, influencing feelings, emotions and inter-relationships within the environment.

INDIVIDUAL TOES AND THEIR MEANINGS

Third Toe/The Doing Toe

Rebounds thoughts regarding activity, personal achievements, self actualisation and inner control.

Fourth Toe/The Communicating Toe

Demonstrates the impact of thoughts regarding communication, relationships and pleasure.

Little Toe/The Moving Toe
Displays the degree of security of thoughts, influenced by family, upbringing and social belief systems, that affect the expansiveness and freedom of thought. Secure thoughts experience the fullness of life's adventures.

CHARACTERISTICS OF THE TOES

Staying on the balls of the toes
- Each toe pad reflects specific aspects of thought and the impression of those perceptions and ideas.

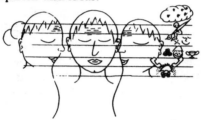

THE DIVISIONS OF TOE PADS RELATED TO THE HEAD

TIPS OF THE TOES

Top of the head reflexes. Space to think.
Reflect clarity of thought, degree of tolerance and amount of space available to play around with and develop ideas.

Flaking skin: Extreme irritability from life getting 'under the skin'. Perfectionists who prefer to complete tasks themselves to their own perceived high standard. Acceptance of the self makes others more tolerable.

Hard skin: Hides or protects true thoughts, ideas and perceptions. Conceals irritability at not being in control.

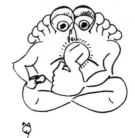

HARD SKIN ON TIPS.
CONCEALING IRRITABILITY

★ *89*

Flaking skin over hard skin: Frustrated at having to suppress and hide personal thoughts. Changing the mind.

Dented: Ideas knocked and not taken seriously.

Horizontal lines across the toes: Think through ideas step by step. Analytical thinker. Apprehensive or perturbed.

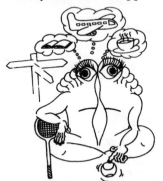

Vertical line(s) down the toe: Divided thoughts. In two minds.

Deep vertical line: Definite change of mind e.g. from one religion to another.

Feint scattered lines: Scatterbrain. Thoughts all over the place!

Prominent toe print: Individualist who identifies well with own ideas.

LINED BIG TOE. DIVIDED THOUGHTS

Superimposed fingerprint: Thoughts, ideas and perception under the influence of others. Cannot think for the self. Emulating another.

Restricted and narrower: Feeling pressurised, as though constrained by a tight band, restricting the ability to think for the self.

IMMEDIATELY BELOW THE TIPS

The temple reflexes. The expression of ideas, thoughts and perceptions. Ideas, thoughts and perceptions leave their mark on this part of the toe.

Horizontal lines across the toes: Concern, worry and anxiety.

Vertical lines down the toe: Displeasure, disapproval or profound thought.

Deep vertical line: Definite concern or deeply pensive.

Feint scattered lines: Fleeting fears and anxieties.

FEINT SCATTERED LINES. FLEETING FEARS AND ANXIETIES

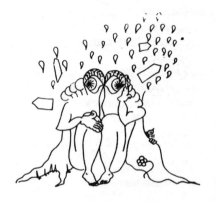

One man's stress is another man's challenge!

UPPER CENTRAL PART OF TOE PAD

Eye reflexes. Feelings and emotions, especially those of unconditional love.

The soul's true thoughts, feelings and emotions are mirrored onto this part of the toe pad, to provide insight. Intuitive universal thoughts are naturally absorbed into the body through the mind's eye. Eyes 'look up' for inspiration and bright ideas!

Vibrant: Balanced, intuitive and able to see and think clearly. Excellent foresight and lively anticipation.

Hard skin: Wearing blinkers and blocking intuition. Prevents seeing and acknowledging the truth.

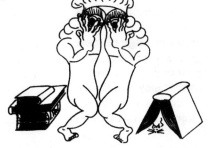

WEARING BLINKERS!
TURNING A BLIND EYE!

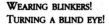

Hard ridge of skin: Divided perceptions and sees two points of view. Displays certain beliefs but keeps true thoughts to the self. Often spiritual souls.

Swollen: Overwhelming fervour and passionate views. Blocking insight.

Resistance: Not wanting to see other points of view and inhibiting intuition.

Hardened hollows: Lack of interest or fearful of seeing the truth about the self.

View the past by filtering it through a different set of lenses, especially if the past is a liability rather than an asset!

LOWER CENTRAL PAD

Ears, cheek and nose reflexes. Active thoughts for self-actualisation.

Sensitive interpretation of ideas and effective instigation of thoughts depends on:

- attention to and comprehension of what is heard (ear reflexes),
- curiosity, inquisitiveness and assertiveness (nose reflexes),
- audacity and impudence (cheek reflexes)!

OUTER   INNER   OUTER

INNER AND OUTER JOINTS OF TOES

Corn on outer edge of toes:
'Turns a deaf ear' to guard against hearing emotive words that may create mental havoc, internal conflict and discomfort. Disregards inner voice.

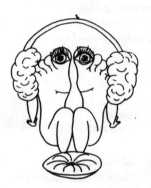

CORNS ON THE OUTER EDGE.
'TURNING A DEAF EAR'

Dent over cheek reflexes: Boldness, impudence and confidence bashed. Threatening relationships knock the enjoyment out of life.
Sunken inner joint: Little or no perceived self-worth.
Swollen outer joint: Head exploding with all that is heard!

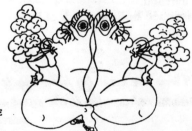

SWOLLEN OUTER JOINT. BLOWING A FUSE

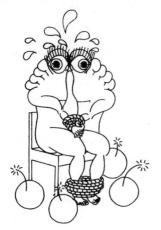

Itching over inner joint: Itching for recognition.

Swollen inner joint: Seeking personal acknowledgement. Feeling emotionally out of control.

Lined inner joint: Number of times self-esteem has been threatened.

SWOLLEN INNER JOINT. EMOTIONALLY THREATENED!

Hard skin over inner joint: Prevents the nose from being knocked out of joint and protects self-esteem. Emotionally vulnerable. Ultra-sensitive. Deep need for recognition.

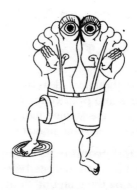

HARD SKIN OVER INNER JOINT: 'NOSE KNOCKED OUT OF JOINT!'

By stilling the whirling of the mind it is easier to see and hear more clearly!

IMMEDIATELY BELOW PREVIOUS REFLEX

Mouth reflexes. Articulate thoughts exchanged to enhance relationships.

A wise man speaks from the heart.
A fool says what he thinks he should say!

Pleasure derived from making decisions (teeth reflexes) and the satisfaction acquired from chewing over, talking through and sharing ideas (mouth reflexes) help to decide which thoughts are of value and those that need to be dismissed. All this is mirrored by the mouth reflexes.

Well-communicated thoughts enhance relationships, whereas being tongue-tied inhibits the flow of words.

Swollen: Mouth full of un-uttered words. Keeping the mouth shut and withholding decisions.

Hard skin: Not able to speak up for the self.

Flaking skin: Frustrated and irritated at not being able to interact openly and honestly. Having words put into the mouth.

THE BASE OF THE TOE PAD

Jaw and chin reflexes. Sound decisions and mobility of thought.

Once I was indecisive, now I am not so sure!

Belief in thoughts, ideas and perceptions provide the confidence to put ideas into practice for growth, expansion and progress. The mobility of the jawline indicates the degree of security perceived and is reflected onto the line at the base of the toe pad.

Hard and prominent: Uncertain about decisions but determined to stand by them despite being in a perceivably prejudiced society! 'Sticking the chin out' through sheer perseverance, single-mindedness or obstinacy.

Hard skin: Extremely insecure and uncertain. Relentlessly adamant and determined. Sticking to decisions despite the opposition! Long-standing resentment. Suppressed need for revenge. Gritting the teeth!

HARD SKIN OVER JAW REFLEX.
DETERMINATION OR OBSTINACY!

Flaking skin over hard skin: Irritated at having to justify and defend thoughts and ideas, or at being considered obstinate!

Dent: Decisions knocked. Teeth knocked out!

We feel secure with those who agree with us,
but we grow with those that don't!

THE UPPER ASPECT OF THE TOES

Cranium and back of the head reflexes. Shield, protect and back thoughts, ideas and decisions.

Corns: Guard personal ideas and prevent them from being trampled and stamped upon. Hard skin safeguards individual thoughts and decisions from total submission to the beliefs of others.

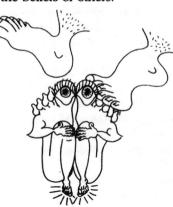

Above the toe joint: Shield ideas, concepts and decisions.

Below the toe joint: Defends the expression of ideas and provides extra backing.

On the sides of the toes: Barrier to listening to the inner voice.

PREVENT IDEAS AND DECISIONS FROM BEING TRAMPLED ON

Silence often has the loudest voice!

Reflexology footnote

✳ STRETCH TOES APART, AS FAR AS COMFORTABLY POSSIBLE, TO EASE PRESSURE ON THE MIND AND MAKE SPACE TO THINK! ESPECIALLY GOOD DURING PARTICULARLY DEMANDING PERIODS!

THE INFLUENCE OF THE SUBCONSCIOUS MIND ON THE STATURE OF THE TOES

A wise man alters his life by altering his attitude!

Well-spaced toes: Open-minded and actively search universal truth. Plenty of space for thoughts and inspiration.

Well-proportioned, flexible toes: Well adjusted, full of vitality with an active mind and a balanced approach to life. Think clearly.

Rigid toes: Definite, unbending views. Consuming ambition and need to dominate. Obstinate and deeply insecure.

Upstanding toes: Able to stand up to own ideas and face the world with confidence.

Toes all in a line: Solid, consistent, even thoughts.

Uneven toes: Inconsistent thinking. Up and down!

Overlapping toes: No room for own ideas. Lack freedom of thought. Overriding own ideas!

Crushed toes: Dominated, smothered and stifled.

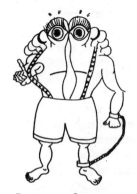

RIGID TOES: SET BELIEF SYSTEMS!

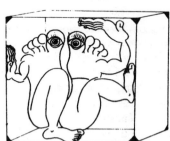

OVERLAPPING TOES:
'NO SPACE TO THINK'

Squashed, cramped toes: Thinking cramped and moulded to conform to rigid beliefs, leading to insecurity, frustration and narrow-mindedness. No time or space to pursue own ideas or be an individual. Feels dominated and subservient. Single-minded.

Toes sunken into their socket:
Given in to the constant hammering of ideas, thoughts or perceptions. Lacking a firm basis.

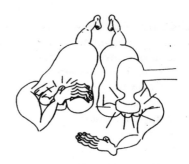

SUNKEN TOES: IDEAS HAMMERED INTO THE GROUND!

Twisted toes: Turn away from acknowledging the truth and looking to others for reassurance.

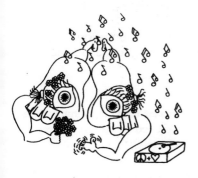

Sloping toes: Off track, insecure and inflexible. Not able to think for the self. Shifts thoughts to please others. Reluctant to stand up to others for fear of ridicule. Ideas are perceived to be too way out for general acceptance!

SLOPING TOE: SHIFTS WAY OUT THOUGHTS TO CONFORM!

Toe stands alone: Thoughts separated to retain their individuality. Needs space to think.

Toes that stand back: Holding back ideas. Shy and withdrawn. Stands back to observe. Not prepared to stand in line! Stand-offish!

Toes that push forward: Trying to get ideas across and seeking recognition. Interested, adamant or involved.

Concealed toe: Shy, withdrawn and hiding in the hope of not being noticed. Lacks confidence and is over-sensitive.

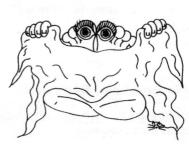

CONCEALED TOE: SHY, SELF-CONSCIOUS AND WITHDRAWN

Bent toes: Fear responsibility or failure. Frightened to face up to having own ideas. Bending to other belief systems. Hanging head in embarrassment, disappointment or shame. Selfconscious.

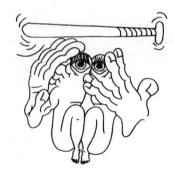

BENT TOE: 'UNABLE TO FACE THE WORLD'

Toes with a rigid bend at the joint: Does not want to see other points of view. Resisting others' belief systems, but ending up off-course anyway!

Toes that bow over their necks: Bowing into submission. Not trusting intuition. 'Bull in a china shop'. Trying to grasp an idea, hold onto a decision or curling in glee.

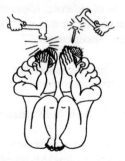

Knocked toes: Personal beliefs knocked or battered. Feel rejected.

KNOCKED TOES: THOUGHTS AND IDEAS BATTERED

Suppressed toes: Ideas and thoughts dominated and overruled. Individuality subdued into conformity.

Hammer toes: Ideas hammered and knocked. Severe intellectual tension and distress interfere with the thinking process. Extremely insecure.

Reflexology footnote

✱ ROTATE EACH TOE INDIVIDUALLY, ANTICLOCKWISE, THEN CLOCKWISE, TO LOOSEN NECK TENSION.

Crooked toes: Modifies and adapts thinking to please others, but the discomfort encourages devious thoughts.

Knobbed toes: Trying to break free from restrictive thoughts.

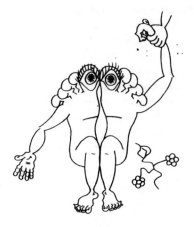

CROOKED TOES: 'ADAPTING TO INAPPROPRIATE BELIEF SYSTEMS'

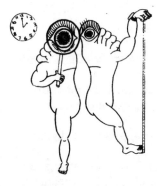

KNOTTED TOES: 'PRECISELY SO!'

Knotted toes: Analytical, precise, calculating decisions and thoughts. Tied up with own way of thinking.

Webbed toes: Thoughts interdependent on one another for extra backup and the two-way exchange of energy.

Gangrenous toes: Mortification of ideas and concepts. Self-denial, humiliation or deeply hurt. No longer nourished with vibrancy and energy.

Amputated toes: Subconsciously severing of ideas and own way of thinking.

THE INFLUENCE OF THE SUBCONSCIOUS MIND ON THE TOE PADS

Vibrant and balanced: Intuitively spontaneous and creative.

Well-rounded pads: Space to throw around ideas, think through and reflect upon perceptions. Enjoys exercising the mind and thinking for the self. Intellectuals or those who think in a 'round about' way.

Bulging pads: Bursting with
unexpressed ideas!

Flaccid pads: Giving into
others. Lacking substance.

Square pads: Conformist,
traditionalist, 'fuddy duddy',
stick-in-the-mud! Ideas boxed
in and contained. Like to
have a 'frame of reference'.
Confined thoughts.

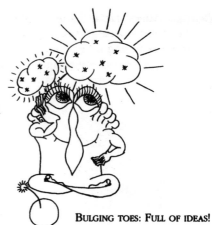

BULGING TOES: FULL OF IDEAS!

Straight, narrow pads: Grasp concepts quickly. Logical mind that
keeps to the straight and narrow. No 'beating about the bush'.
Opinionated!

Pointed pads: Go straight to the point. Direct approach. If slightly
rounded, the blow is softened.

Funnel-shaped pads: Flat- or square-topped. Thoughts easily access
universal knowledge. Deep inner understanding. Often dreamers,
artists, musicians, psychics and esoteric practitioners with a natural
ability to channel.

Elegant and dainty pads: Soft, gentle, sophisticated thoughts and
ideas.

Thick skin over pads: Masking
true thoughts, ideas and
identity. Concealing personal
perceptions.

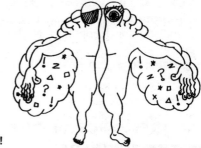

THICK-SKINNED TOE PADS! EXTRA-
PROTECTIVE TOWARDS OWN THOUGHTS!

'Plastic' covering over pad: Covering up false thoughts. 'Jekyll and
Hyde' existence. Lost touch with own reality.

Superimposed covering over pad: Putting on a front, masking true
thoughts or two-faced. Thinking on two levels, in two minds.

Dented, pitted pads: Thoughts perceivably knocked and ridiculed due to uncertainty, insecurity or from feeling threatened e.g. a foreigner having difficulty in thinking in an alien manner.

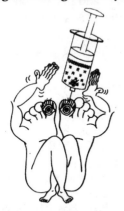

Shrivelled pads: Recoils and withdraws. Cringes with fear and backs off. Ability to think for the self is diminished.

Flattened pads: Keep 'falling flat on the face'. Trip the self up with own thoughts and ideas. Monotonous, unexciting and demotivated perceptions.

SHRIVELLED TOE: DIMINISHED THOUGHTS

GENERAL MARKINGS ON THE WHOLE TOE PAD

Vertical lines down centre: Divided thoughts. Split down the middle. Can see two points of view.

Deep vertical line: Deeply affected by a change of mind.

Prominent toe print: Individualist who identifies well with own ideas.

Superimposed fingerprint: Thoughts, ideas and decisions influenced by others.

Long raised line down side of the toe: Feeling divided. Wearing a mask. Putting on a brave face, or two-faced.

White pockets beneath the skin: Collection of inflamed, angry thoughts that fester beneath the surface.

Corns: Protects toes from being trodden on and having personal views and ideas stamped out. Prevents total submission to other belief systems, to retain own identity.

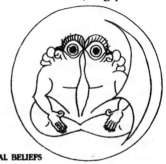

CORNS: PROTECTING PERSONAL BELIEFS

THE INTER-RELATIONSHIP OF THE TOES

The relationship between toes provides insight as to the harmony between individual thoughts, ideas, concepts and perceptions. There are several types of relationship and, in some cases, more than one may apply:

Supporting: One or both toes prop up and encourage one another.

Squashing: Crushing or crowding out ideas.

Knocking: One or both toes criticise and inhibit thoughts and decisions of one another!

Overlapping: One toe ignores or overrides the perceptions of the other.

Hiding: Keep ideas and thoughts out of sight. Conceal true thoughts behind the concepts of the shielding toes.

Resting: One or both toes rely on the approval and support of the other.

Smooth indentations either side: Ideas rub up against one another.

Between big and second toes: intellectual thoughts conflict with personal opinion.

Between second and third toes: ideas about activity go against grain of personal concepts or 'ruffle the feathers' when thinking of various pursuits!

Between third and fourth toes: active thoughts create friction within the perceptive realm of communication and relationships.

Between fourth and fifth toes: concepts of security and mobility clash with those of communication and relationships. (See Appendix III.)

THE EMOTIONAL ASPECT OF THE TOES

The position of various colourings and different textures on the toes reflects the emotional aspect of thought, with continual fluctuations mirroring mood swings.

Vibrant and flesh-coloured: Alert, active mind filled with enthusiasm.

White toe: Drained of energy and too exhausted to think.

Pockets of white beneath skin's surface: Inflamed thoughts and ideas accumulate and simmer beneath the surface.

Blue toe: Painful or injured thoughts and a bruised ego!

Red toe: Embarrassed, angry or frustrated at the possibility of ideas, principles and beliefs being questioned or threatened.

Yellow toe: Resentful, critical views with jaundiced perceptions.

Green toe: Envious thoughts.

Wrinkled toe: Continual concern and perpetual worry.

Flaking skin: Extremely irritated at not being allowed to think for the self.

Large arrogant toe: Likes to dominate and be in total control.

*Attitude is a state of mind,
if you don't like it,
change it!*

Reflexology footnotes

* DURING A READING OR TREATMENT, TOE CHARACTERISTICS AND RELATIONSHIPS CHANGE AS THOUGHTS RESPOND TO SHIFTS IN CONSCIOUSNESS AND CHANGING EMOTIONS. FOR EXAMPLE, BENT TOES STRAIGHTEN, SHY TOES COME FORWARD AND SO ON, AS TENSION RELEASES ITS GRIP ON THE WHOLE MUSCULATURE.

* BABIES OFTEN CURL OR EXTEND TOES, WHILST SUCKLING AT THE BREAST, FROM COMPLETE ECSTASY OF SUCCUMBING TO PHYSICAL PLEASURE AND WILLINGLY SURRENDERING TO THE CARE OF OTHERS! BABIES' AND CHILDREN'S TOES CHANGE DRAMATICALLY, AS THEY INCREASINGLY CONFORM TO RIGID PARENTAL AND SOCIAL BELIEF SYSTEMS, DEPRIVING THEM OF THE CAPACITY TO DREAM IN AN IMAGINARY 'MAKE-BELIEVE' WORLD.

* TOE MASSAGE AND MANIPULATION CLEARS THE MIND AND CREATES A BRIGHTER UNDERSTANDING.

THE SOLE PERSPECTIVE

Every day is a new day with new opportunities and new experiences!

The lower, protective surfaces of the feet, the soles, provide a firm but flexible foundation from which to grow and develop. As bases, they provide a deep understanding of the self, others and life.

Solid, female, negative, *yin* energies, from Mother earth, are absorbed into the body, through the soles, to intermingle with light, male, positive, *yang* energies of the sun, drawn in by the rest of the body to provide a healthy balance of vibrant life-forces.

Soles are remarkable sources of precise information, and reflect how ethereal thoughts are physically manifested on the material plane.

Predominantly large toes belong to the 'thinkers', whilst predominantly large soles belong to the 'doers'!

The right sole reflects past impressions, whilst the left sole is more impressed by the present.

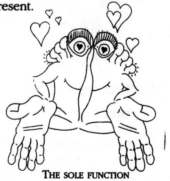

THE SOLE FUNCTION

The sole's sole purpose is to support the soul!

CHARACTERISTICS OF THE SOLE

Well proportioned: Well balanced. Assimilates abstract knowledge and applies it with ease on the physical plane.

Broad and solid: Industrious, honest and loyal.

Broad and supple: Spontaneous and grasps concepts well to put them into action. These 'kind soles' enjoy doing things, especially for others.

Prominently large: The need to survive in the physical world takes precedence over all else. Physical actions dominate intellectual reasoning. Common in those who have had to survive despite the odds.

Hard and coarse: Feeling vulnerable, so builds up a resistance leading to inflexibility and stubbornness. True thoughts and feelings are concealed.

Firm and supple: Refined sentiments and a high integrity with a constant need to improve.

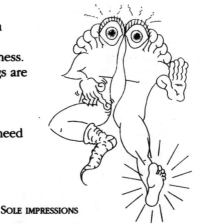

SOLE IMPRESSIONS

SIGNIFICANCE OF THE VARIOUS SECTIONS OF THE SOLE

The position of impressions, marks and colourings on the soles of the feet reflect specific aspects of thoughts, ideas and perceptions when put into practice.

POSITION	BENEATH THE BIG	BENEATH THE SECOND	BENEATH THE THIRD	BENEATH THE FOURTH	BENEATH THE LITTLE
	Thoughts	Feelings	Actions	Communications	Security and mobility
ON THE BALLS OF THE FEET	Space for the self	The effect of personal perceptions	The active manifestation of sentiment	Emotional feelings regarding relationships	Space for the family and room for expansion

POSITION	BENEATH THE BIG	BENEATH THE SECOND	BENEATH THE THIRD	BENEATH THE FOURTH	BENEATH THE LITTLE
ON THE UPPER INSTEP	The actualisation of the soul's purpose	The confidence for personal activities	Energy and enthusiasm to put ideas into practice	Effective communication for good working relationships	Trust own concepts to be expansively manifested
ON THE LOWER INSTEP	Effective communication between the soul and the universe for balanced relationships	Ability to give and take of the self with ease	Active exchange of life-forces	Attraction and rejection of relationships for inner harmony	Sufficiently secure to let go of the old and attract the new for the expansion of life
ON THE HEEL	A firm basis for the soul to achieve its full potential	Basic understanding and trust of the self to move ahead	Appropriate actions spurn the individual on to greater accomplishments	The flow of life eases progress and enhances relationships along the way	A secure foundation to venture out and experience the unknown

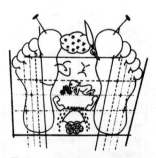

THE DIVISIONS ON THE SOLES
AND THEIR MEANINGS

SOUL TO SOLE

'Sole' sounds like 'soul', linking the soul to the earth plane, and sole characteristics are outward expressions of the inner soul. The soul, as the immaterial part of man, contains vital energy for moral and spiritual growth and understanding.

Sole means one, but the two soles signify the duality required for the balance of life, e.g. male/female, positive/negative, dark/light, and so on.

The right sole reflects past connections down through the ages, whilst the left sole is the link to the future and all it holds, which ultimately depends on the way in which the path of life has been trodden.

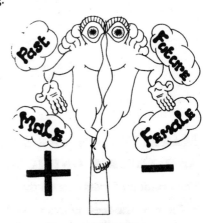

SOLES: THE BALANCE OF LIFE

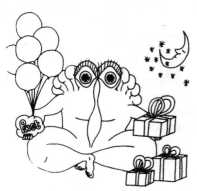

PAST, PRESENT AND FUTURE

An anagram of the word sole is lose. Soles will lose their way when they deviate from their soul's purpose.

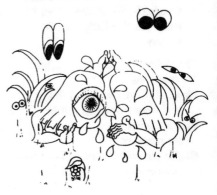

Ultimately all souls aim to lose the need to manifest themselves physically on earth and, although part of the whole, this process is dependent on individual progress, hence the sole experience of life.

LOST SOLES

★ *57*

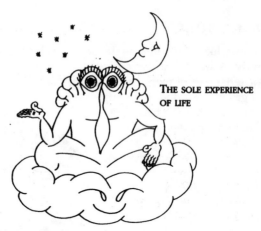

THE SOLE EXPERIENCE
OF LIFE

MARKINGS ON THE SOLES OF THE FEET AND THEIR SIGNIFICANCE

The position of markings on the soles of the feet is meaningful:

- **Balls of the feet:** Emotions within the environment related to feelings of self-worth.
- **Upper insteps:** Activity and enthusiasm for life.
- **Lower insteps:** Communications and relations.
- **Heels:** Basis for stability and mobility.
- **Beneath the big toe:** Intellectual influence.
- **Beneath the second toe:** Relating to the self.
- **Beneath the third toe:** Effect on activities.
- **Beneath the fourth toe:** Social interaction.
- **Beneath the little toe:** Security and space within the family and society.

Flexible: Adapts easily to life's situations.

Flaccid: Gives in too quickly and very impressionable.

Firm: Constrained, orderly and set manner.

Rigid: Insecure, inflexible, adamant and unbending.

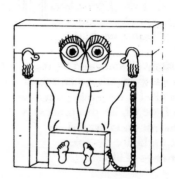

RIGIDITY: UNBENDING VIEWS

Swollen: Weighed down and overburdened with unshed tears.

Swellings: Areas of congested, unresolved emotions.

Wrinkled: Extreme concern and anxiety.

Flattened: Meeting resistance and drained of vitality. Everything falls flat!

Hard skin: Shields, protects and conceals.

Horizontal lines: Divide or cut up, reducing life into smaller manageable-sized pieces. Step-by-step approach.

Vertical lines: The divisions of life that keep two areas separate.

Deep fissures: Detach two sections from one another.

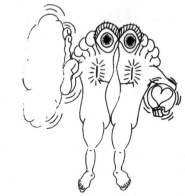

DEEP FISSURE: CUT UP AND DIVIDED

Crossed lines: Crossroads requiring a decision to be made.

A cross: A cross to bear.

Boxed lines: Certain aspects of life boxed off and contained.

Circular lines: Going around in circles or working around a situation!

Random lines: Confusion with a whirlwind, or sometimes a volcanic, effect.

Stars: Well-blessed. Universal help available.

Dagger lines: Emotionally stabbed.

Blisters: Friction and rubbing up against resistance.

Brown/black marks and freckles: Deep hurts.

Block of differing colour: A whole section kept in 'the dark', separated or blocked off.

Prominent blood vessels: Old emotions and burdens subconsciously emerging.

White accumulations beneath the skin: Suppressed emotions festering beneath the surface.

Paw or hoof mark: Animal making an impression.

Horse shoe: Good luck!

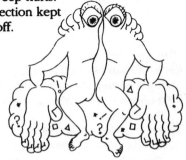

WHITE POCKETS UNDER SKIN: INTENSE EMOTIONS SUPPRESSED!

* 59

The Big Toe and its Related Parts, the Necks of the Toes

THE BIG TOE – THE THINKING TOE

The head and brain reflexes

Symbolises: Intellectual
thoughts.
Qualities: Intuition and
spirituality.
Element: Ether, the spacious
quality of thoughts.
Colour: Indigo/violet, the
highest colour vibration.
Connections: All toes and the
nervous system.
Related to: The thumb and toe necks.
Direct reflexes: On the toe pad:
Head, face, brain, pituitary
gland, pineal gland, thyroid
gland, sensory organs and neck.
Indirect reflexes: On top of
the toe: Cranium, midbrain
and cervical vertebrae.

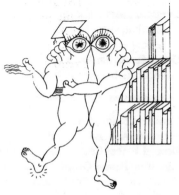

THE THINKING TOE

Optimism is an intellectual choice!

The main reflexes for the head and brain rebound onto the fleshy
pads of both big toes to reflect the state of mind constantly. Continual
thought patterns, as well as the subtle influences of the subconscious
and unconscious brains, leave their mark on the big toe pads.

Big toes interact intuitively and astutely with the environment,
whereas resistance to the flow of life deflects them, causing them to
bend and generally displace the other toes.

The right big toe carries past impressions, whilst the left big toe
reflects present perceptions.

CHARACTERISTICS OF THE BIG TOE

- A straight, upstanding, flexible big toe expresses expansive thoughts with confidence and humour. It exudes confidence, optimism, independence and influence.
- The natural length of the big toe corresponds to the potential level of awareness. A good-sized, long big toe enthusiastically seeks spiritual enlightenment whilst a shorter, stubby big toe is anchored to the perceived security of the physical world. The latter tends to be more impressionable and impulsive.
- The shape and size of the pad on the big toe show aptitude for thought and space available for playing around with ideas.
- The neck of the big toe indicates capacity for thoughts to be put into practice and the consequences of that activity.
- The outline, created by the pads of the two big toes, placed side by side, closely resembles the shape of the face.

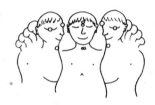

THE BIG TOE AND ITS RELATIONSHIP WITH
THE NECKS OF THE TOES

PARTS RELATED TO THE BIG TOE

Head: Facilitates the ability to get ahead with clarity of thought and many ideas.

Face: Has the confidence to face the world and expose personal perceptions.

Brain: The brains behind the thoughts to ignite ideas.

Pituitary gland: Controls and balances emotions to calm the mind.

Pineal gland: Provides insight and intuition to draw on universal knowledge.

Thyroid gland: Allows space for self expression.

Sensory organs: Sensitively pick up impulses and interpret them appropriately.

Neck: Two-way channel for the expressions of life. 'Get it in the neck' by contradicting others.

THE INFLUENCE OF THE SUBCONSCIOUS MIND ON THE BIG TOE

(See also general toe characteristics page 61)

It's not what we think, but how we think it!

Flexible: Goes with the flow. Confident, adaptable and progresses with ease. Considerate. Makes headway.

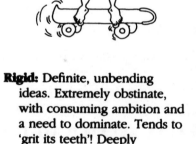

A FLEXIBLE BIG TOE: BALANCED, CONSIDERATE AND PROGRESSIVE

Rigid: Definite, unbending ideas. Extremely obstinate, with consuming ambition and a need to dominate. Tends to 'grit its teeth'! Deeply insecure.

RIGID BIG TOE:
SET THOUGHTS AND IDEAS

Trust intuition to show the way!

Band around top: Thoughts restricted and confined due to outside pressure. Pressure cooker effect.

Change your mind and change your life!

Extra extension: Thoughts reach out towards an extended plane.

Split in two: Ffyona Campbell's big toes apparently split into two during her trek across Africa, possibly indicating that she was in two minds as to whether to continue. In order to survive and remain sane, she needed to divide and separate her thoughts.

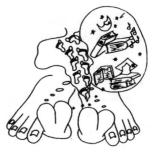

BIG TOE SPLIT IN TWO:
IN TWO MINDS – LITERALLY!

THE NECKS OF THE TOES

Neck and throat reflexes

Symbolises: The two-way exchange of life-forces for the intermingling of ethereal and physical forces.
Qualities: Flexibility and the free exchange of energies, easing interaction.
Elements: Ether/air, uninhibited space for interchange.
Colour: Turquoise blue.
Connection: Nervous system.
Related to: All the toes, especially the big toe, and the thumb.
Direct reflexes: Underneath the feet: Throat, oesophagus, trachea and larynx.
Indirect reflexes: On the upper aspect of the feet: Back of neck, and tonsils.

Reflexology footnotes

✱ PREDOMINANT USE OF THE THUMB DURING REFLEXOLOGY, GIVING PARTICULAR ATTENTION TO THE TOES, ESPECIALLY THE BIG TOE, STIMULATES THE BRAIN REFLEXES, THEREBY RAISING THE LEVEL OF SUBCONSCIOUS THOUGHT, FACILITATING MEMORY, CLEARING THE MIND AND RELIEVING ANXIETY.

✱ TO EASE NECK AND NERVOUS TENSION, PULL EACH PAIR OF TOES SIMULTANEOUSLY, WITH THE BODY LYING FLAT, THEN ROTATE EACH TOE INDIVIDUALLY, ANTICLOCKWISE AND THEN CLOCKWISE.

The head and body are physically connected via the neck, which facilitates the two-way exchange of the energies of life. The way in which these vital forces are channelled into and out of the body is mirrored onto the necks of the toes.

The working of the mind (toes) is manifested in the body (soles) through the neck (toe necks) generating further thoughts (toes) and on-going activity (soles). Each toe neck expresses the exchange of specific life-forces.

THE EXPRESSIONS OF THE INDIVIDUAL NECKS OF THE TOES

Neck of the big toe: The intellectual, intuitive and spiritual exchange of thoughts and actions.

Neck of the second toe: The honest expression of the self and unconditional love.

Neck of the third toe: The energetic reciprocation of thoughts and actions.

Neck of the fourth toe: The pleasurable interaction of relationships through good communications throughout the whole.

Neck of the little toe: The mobile expression and exchange of life's adventures based on security, family and movement.

THE INFLUENCE OF THE SUBCONSCIOUS MIND ON THE NECKS OF THE TOES

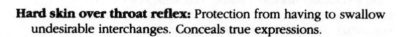

Swollen throat reflex: 'Hard to swallow' aspects of life causing a lump of congested emotions. Holding back unshed tears and unexpressed feelings. Inner crying.

SWOLLEN THROAT REFLEX

Hard skin over throat reflex: Protection from having to swallow undesirable interchanges. Conceals true expressions.

Ridge of hard skin: Division between the way life energies are exchanged and would like to be expressed!

Wrinkled throat reflex:
Extreme anxiety and concern at swallowing so many unpalatable situations, or exhaustion from trying to express personal ideas. Aware of the need to give and take, but does not always know how!

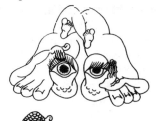

WRINKLED THROAT REFLEX

Vertical lines across throat reflex: Strained exchange or 'compartmentalising' life's expressions.

Vertical crevice across throat reflex: 'Cut the throat' due to difficult interaction.

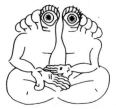

HORIZONTAL LINES ACROSS THROAT REFLEX

Horizontal line across throat reflex: Choked and restrained. Take things in or express the self little by little, step by step.

One line across the centre: Prepared to give and take a certain amount.

Two lines divide the neck into three: Difficulty in intermingling life's expressions and so a vacuum separates the two.

Jester's collar: Life's expressions, especially the difficult ones, are dealt with with humour.

Drawn throat: Throttled as though a rope is around the throat.

Scarring over throat reflex: Wound from having had the throat slit.

Corns on top of the throat reflex: Prevent personal expressions from succumbing to perceived threats.

Cut between the toes: Divided expressions cut off from one another. (For greater understanding see the significance of each toe and its meaning on page 38.)

Cut at the base of the neck reflex: Slash the throat because unable to put ideas into practice. 'Stopped in their tracks'. Divorcing the self from the physical world.

Big toe – swelling at base of neck (Thyroid gland reflexes): Resents giving priority to the needs of others, leaving little or no time for the self.

Big toe – hard skin at base of neck (Thyroid gland reflexes): Protects and guards time and space for the self.

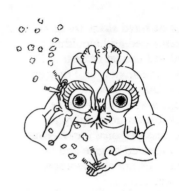

SWOLLEN THYROID REFLEXES:
NO TIME FOR THE SELF!

Big toe – flaking skin over the hard skin at neck base: Irritable from having to conceal resentment at having to run around others.

THE LENGTH OF THE TOE NECKS

The length of toe necks conveys the potential for expressive creativity. The space encourages universal thoughts to mingle with solid physical vibrations, to provide balance for self-development and self-expression.

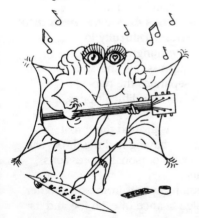

Long necks on all toes: Considerable creative talent. Often with the 'head in the clouds'. Easily access universal creativity. Common in artists and musicians.

LONG NECKS ON TOES:
HEAD IN THE CLOUDS!

Short necks: Practical approach to life with feet firmly on the ground.

No necks: No space for self expression. Whole thrust either intellectual or physical. Not speaking up for the self. Holding back.

Long necks on second and third toes and shorter necks on fourth and fifth toes: Equally balanced creativity and practical application.

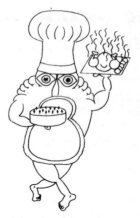

NO NECKS ON TOES: FEET FIRMLY ON THE GROUND!

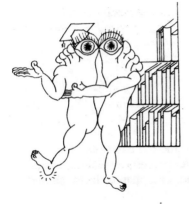

WEBBED TOES: POTENTIAL GENIUS!

Webbed necks, joining second and third toes: Potential genius. Self-esteem depends on career and activities.

The Second Toe and its Related Parts, the Ball of the Foot, the Heart and Solar Plexus Reflexes

THE SECOND TOE – THE FEELING TOE

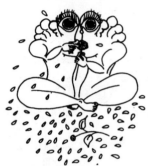

THE FEELING TOE

Symbolises: Thoughts regarding personal perceptions of the self.

Qualities: Individuality and unconditional love.

Element: Air space for the interchange of feelings and emotions.

Colour: Turquoise green.

Connection: Respiratory system.

Related to: The index finger, the ego, and the ball of the foot.

Direct reflexes: On the soles of the feet: Chest, respiratory system, breasts, thyroid gland, thymus gland, oesophagus, heart, shoulders and solar plexus.

Indirect reflexes: On the top of the foot: Upper back, upper arms and knees.

Cooperation and harmony between individuals is only possible when there is cooperation and harmony within the self?

The air characteristic of the second toe and respiratory tract encourages expansiveness and adaptability to ever-changing environmental conditions.

Individual response to outer events depends on current emotional states, as well as feelings of self-worth. Those who feel good about themselves go with the flow of life, regardless of circumstances, making the most of each and every situation.

Poor self-esteem hampers individual progress, even in the most conducive surroundings, leading to frustration, discontent and poor self-worth.

The right second toe reflects past impressions of self-esteem, whilst the left second toe reflects present thoughts and feelings.

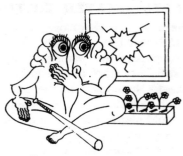

FEELINGS EASILY HURT

If we long for kindness, we need to be kind; if we yearn for the truth, we must be true to ourselves, for what we give of ourselves is always reflected back.

CHARACTERISTICS OF THE SECOND TOE

Become the most positive person you know!

- A proud, upstanding second toe feels good about itself, thinks clearly, integrates well and exchanges ideas with ease.
- The natural length of the second toe conveys potential capacity for personal success. The longer the toe, the greater the ability to guide and instil confidence in others.
- The shape and size of the toe pad on the second toe, indicate potential for social integration.
- The neck of the second toe permits self-expression.
- Long second toes are particularly common on Arians, Leos and Capricorns!

THE SECOND TOE AND ITS RELATIONSHIP
TO THE BALL OF THE FEET

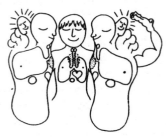

Parts related to the second toe

Chest: Feelings kept close to chest burden the whole. Getting it 'off the chest' takes a 'weight off the mind'. Fearful emotions are suppressed by breath and contained within the chest cavity.

Respiratory tract: Intense emotions immediately affect respiration.

Breasts: Nurturing, from the time of conception, and nurturing of the self, determine feelings and emotions and interaction within society.

Thyroid gland: Time spent on personal expression affects the ability to relate true sentiments.

Thymus gland: Feelings of self-confidence and self-worth affect inter-relationships within the surroundings.

Oesophagus: The peristaltic movements of digestion are immediately influenced by emotions. Anger and frustration speed up the rippling movement, whereas sadness and depression slow it down.

Heart: As the centre of love, types of emotion determine heart functioning.

Shoulders: Shoulders responsibility and takes the weight off the rest of the body. Too much emotion weighs the whole down with perceived burdens.

Upper back: Lovingly supports all feelings and provides a firm backing.

Upper arms: Open wide to embrace affectionately, or folded to cut off the outside world or to keep feelings close to the chest.

Solar plexus: If in control, good feelings are experienced.

The effect of the subconscious mind on the second toe

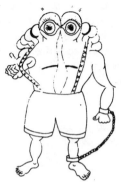

Vibrant, upstanding and flexible: Feels good about itself and blends well into any situation.

Rigid: Self-opinionated, assertive, authoritarian. Unbending beliefs in themselves. Relies on personal opinion and egotistical resources. Nothing will change their mind!

RIGID SECOND TOE: ADAMANT IDEAS AND PERCEPTIONS

The ego misleads the mind into believing that it is what it would like to be rather than what it really is!

Straight: Stands up to own feelings and exchanges ideas confidently.
Small: Lacks nurturing.
Insignificant: Insecure and lacks confidence. Fears of being inadequate. Feels submissive and perceives itself as being victimised.
Webbed with third toe: Self-esteem relies on activities or career.

Lead, follow or get out of the way!

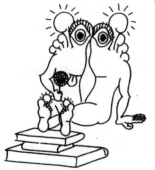

LONG SECOND TOE: A BORN LEADER!

Longer than big toe: Head and shoulders above the rest! Greater vision possible. If inflated, self-opinionated or filled with selfish thoughts, subjugates the intellect. Likes to be seen to be in charge. Potential for outstanding leadership qualities by instilling confidence in others. (Check that the second toe does not appear longer because the big toe is sunken.) Common on Capricorns, Arians and Leos!

Ridge of hard skin down the centre pad: Shields the self from seeing or acknowledging true self worth.

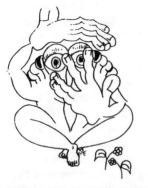

RIDGED SECOND TOE: DENYING PERSONAL WORTH

Trust and believe in yourself, you are all you have!

THE BALL OF THE FOOT

Chest and breast reflexes

Symbolises: The physical interaction and manifestation of feelings
   and emotions, particularly those of self-esteem and self-worth.
Qualities: Feelings of unconditional love and recognition of the truth.
Element: Air providing space for personal expansion.
Colour: Green.
Related to: The second toe and the index finger.
Direct reflexes: The soles of the feet: Shoulders, respiratory tract,
   heart, chest, breasts, oesophagus, thyroid gland, thymus gland and
   solar plexus.
Indirect reflexes: The top of the foot: Upper back and upper arm.

> *Neither genius nor glory truly reflect the human soul,
> only unconditional love and kindness.*

The chest and breast, reflected onto the rounded balls of the feet
immediately below the toes, provide space for interaction within the
environment. Mind, body and soul sustained by atmospheric energies
from the immediate vicinity, via the respiratory tract, are also nurtured
by the breasts.

Inhaled oxygen revitalises and sustains life, whereas exhaled
carbon dioxide, processed by bodily vibrations, fills the environment
with waves of personal emotions and feelings. Hence, vibes within
the atmosphere being almost electric at times!

Those who feel good about themselves, cherish life and take in
large breaths of appreciation. Conversely, victims feel rejected, have
little or no self-worth, and begrudgingly take in the breath of life.

Feelings of love and joy relax the musculature, making space for
massive volumes of air to fill the whole with positive vibrations. No
matter how favourable the environment, it is the atmosphere,
infiltrated by moods and emotions, that ultimately determines
behaviour. Good news is uplifting and energising, regardless of the
weather, whereas disappointing news can make the sunniest of days
pale into insignificance.

Breathing and the distribution of life-forces are also directly affected by the type of nurturing since conception and care of the self in the present.

The overlapping of chest and breast reflexes demonstrate the influence of nurturing on self-esteem and self-worth, which determines personal interaction with physical surroundings. The balls of the feet, therefore, reflect the physical manifestation of feelings and emotions arising from the thoughts of the second toe. Emotional congestion or of feeling 'up to the neck' with unresolved issues, gives the balls of the feet a 'top heavy' appearance, weighing down the whole.

CHARACTERISTICS OF THE BALL OF THE FOOT

- Firm, pliable, vibrant, flesh-coloured balls feel good about themselves and confidently adapt to and accommodate any situation or environment.

Allow your love to cherish yourself, as well as others!

THE EFFECT OF THE SUBCONSCIOUS MIND ON THE BALL OF THE FOOT

Vibrant and pliable: Takes in the breath of life with love, joy and appreciation. Feels good!

Shoulder reflexes: Carry the load to ease burdens. Great relief is experienced when 'a weight is taken off the shoulders'.

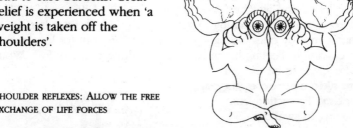

SHOULDER REFLEXES: ALLOW THE FREE EXCHANGE OF LIFE FORCES

Swellings below necks of all toes: Perceived packages of 'responsibility'. Feeling burdened. 'Carrying the world on the shoulders'. Swellings prevent the two way exchange of energy between head and body. The number and position of the swellings indicates the type and quantity of perceived responsibilities, whilst the size is indicative of the enormity of the burden.

Our greatest responsibility is to respond appropriately to every situation, without taking on excess baggage!

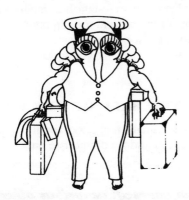

SHOULDER REFLEXES: WEIGHED DOWN WITH RESPONSIBILITIES

Hard skin over the thyroid reflex: Protects or conceals true expressions or time for the self.

Swollen thyroid reflex: A feeling of 'swimming against the tide' leaving little or no time for the self.

Red thyroid reflexes: Anger at inability to express the true self and that there is insufficient time for the self.

Swollen pad: Emotional congestion and unresolved feelings. 'Responsibilities' take up space within the environment. Over-burdened and weighed down by the perceived demands of life.

General swelling: Straining to get in touch with feelings but hampered by outstanding emotions. Reaching out for love and recognition. Feeling hemmed in and wishing to break free. Would like space to be the self.

Hard skin over oesophageal reflex: Protection from having to swallow unpalatable sentiments.

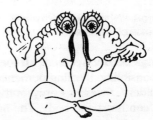

OESOPHAGEAL REFLEX: HARD TO SWALLOW CERTAIN SENTIMENTS

Rigid: Unbending and insecure within the environment.

Hard skin: Provides a shield against perceived criticism or fiercely protects personal identity, time and space. Common on those devoted to caring and nurturing others leaving little or no time to 'catch the breath'.

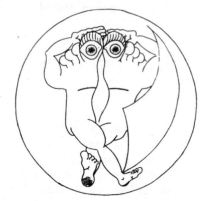

CHEST REFLEXES: HARD SKIN-SHIELDS EMOTIONS

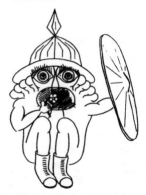

Hard skin over thymus reflex: Disguises vulnerability and protects the self (soul) from perceived verbal, emotional or physical abuse or attack. Continual resistance. Keeping others at bay.

THYMUS REFLEX: HARD SKIN CONCEALS VULNERABILITY

Thumb print over thymus reflex: Under the influence of another who is trying to superimpose their identity onto the soul.

Sunken thymus reflex: Feeling vulnerable and attacked. Poor self-image leads to an inadequate distribution of get up and go, resulting in the abandonment of personal projects and self-destruction of the self. Associated with M.E. and AIDS victims.

Swollen mounds: Denote those who nurture and care for others, and the demands being made on personal space. Too much concern for others can smother them, suffocating the self.

Insignificant or indistinct base line between ball and instep: Others impinging on space, leaving little or no room for the self. Feeling winded or unable to breathe.

Line down the outer edge: Putting on a front. Reluctant to reveal true sensitivity.

Distinctive vertical line or lines: Feeling divided and torn apart by specific aspects of life. Perceived need to lead a double life. For example: living or having lived in two culturally different countries; separating business or schoolife from the home; drastic changes physically due to death, divorce, etc. A vertical line that extends into the instep, means that divided emotions have an impact on activity.

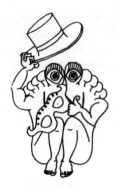

DISTINCT DIVISION: DIVIDED LOYALTIES

Lines drawn to the solar plexus: The number of emotionally dependent people, hampering individual progress.

Swollen sides with protruding bone: Resistance within the environment. Trying to break free. Feel as though the arms are pinned to the sides in a straightjacket, so that life cannot be fully embraced.

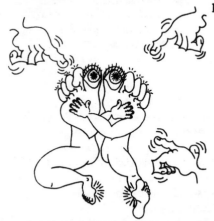

Bunion (*Hallux Valgus*)**:** Angry and inflamed at self-imposed restrictions (if big toe upstanding) or strict upbringing (if big toe bent). Feeling entrapped within the environment due to contained emotions that restrain the self. Would like to break free but too insecure.

BUNION: FEELING CONFINED AND RESTRICTED

Flattened: Vitality drained from having nurtured others to the detriment of the self. (The breast may have been removed due to cancer arising from suppressed resentment at having to keep true feelings and emotions close to the chest.)

Dagger shape pointing down to the hollow immediately below the centre: Feeling emotionally stabbed in the very core of the self.

Dagger shape from the base onto the ball: Breath taken away by some deep emotional dig.

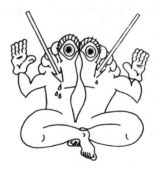

DAGGER SHAPE: FEELING STABBED IN THE CHEST

Deep crevice on lower inside edge over the heart reflex: Effectively separates environmental conditions from draining the love from within, preventing 'hard-heartedness'.

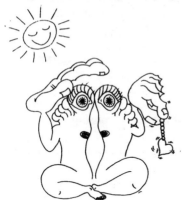

Swollen cardiac sphincter reflex: Difficulty in admitting life's experience. Possible hiatus hernia, indicating severed or ruptured feelings and emotions, placing strain on the heart.

SWOLLEN CARDIAC SPHINCTER: RESTRICTING THE FLOW OF LIFE!

Never deprive anyone of hope – it may be all they have!

Reflexology footnotes

* THE ENERGIES OF THE SECOND FINGER CALM AND REASSURE. THE COOL, BLUE VIBRATIONS SOOTHE, THE GREEN RESONANCE MAKES SPACE, WHILST THE PINK ENERGIES INFUSE THE WHOLE WITH UNCONDITIONAL LOVE.
* MASSAGE AND MANIPULATION OF THE BALLS OF THE FEET CREATE SPACE, EASE INNER TENSION AND BOOST SELF-ESTEEM.

THE HEART REFLEXES

Symbolises: Control of feelings.
Quality: Unconditional love.
Element: Air and fire.
Colour: Green.
Related to: Second and third toes and fingers.
Position on feet: On inner edge where the balls of the feet meet the
  insteps.

The heart, as the centre of love and joy, pulsates vitality and vibrancy
throughout mind, body and soul, keeping them alive with abundant
health. The state of the heart mirrors the mind, feelings, emotions and
moods e.g. kind-hearted, gentle-hearted, hard-hearted, cold-hearted,
and so on.

Loving thoughts soften and expand the heart, allowing love and
joy to flow freely throughout the whole. Thoughts of anger and
frustration constrict the heart, as blood rushes to the face and the
body tenses, depriving cells of essential life-forces and love.

Emotional hurts and abuse, whether given or received, distress the
heart, causing it to harbour resentment and eventually seize up.
Long-term unresolved emotions, fear and deprivation of love create
havoc. The unrelenting tension throughout narrows blood vessels
and creates circulatory, heart and blood disorders, causing
unhappiness and heart dis-ease.

Sickness becomes a focal point of concern and drama in modern-
day society. Reluctance to
improve arises from a fear that
long-overdue love and attention
will be withdrawn, allowing
abandonment and isolation to
return with recovery.

True healing comes from
within and can only occur with
a shift in attitude combined with
unconditional love, first for the
self and then for others.

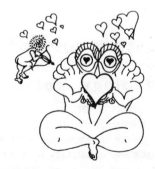

THE HEART REFLEX: THE CENTRE OF
UNCONDITIONAL LOVE

CHARACTERISTICS OF THE HEART REFLEXES

- Heart reflexes are naturally pliable, palpable mounds on the inside edge, immediately below the balls, of both feet.

THE EFFECT OF THE SUBCONSCIOUS MIND ON THE HEART REFLEXES

Swollen: Weighed down by unresolved heartache.

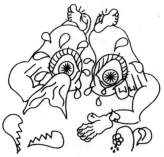

SWOLLEN HEART REFLEX: FILLED WITH ANGUISH AND DESPAIR

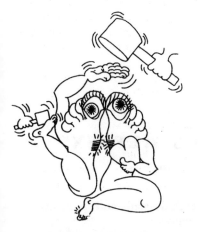

Hardened: Protection against being emotionally wounded or affected by the hurt inflicted on others.

HARDENED HEART: PROTECTING THE SELF AGAINST EMOTIONAL ATTACK

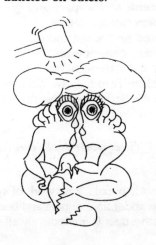

Red with distinct straight or jagged line through it: A broken heart.

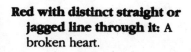

A BROKEN HEART: HEART-BROKEN!

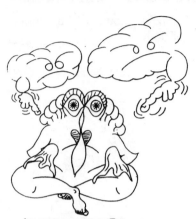

Tiny vessels: A bleeding heart.
Blue, black patches: Deep emotional trauma and hurt.
Hard skin: Protection against being hurt or a means of hiding true feelings of love.

AN INJURED HEART: FEELING EMOTIONALLY BATTERED

THE SOLAR PLEXUS REFLEX

The 'Abdominal Brain' and Centre of Emotions

Symbolises: The centre of emotion.
Qualities: Feeling in control emotionally, physically and spiritually.
Element: Air for space and fire to fuel emotions.
Colour: Golden yellow.
Related to: Second and third toes, index and middle fingers.
Primary connection: The digestive tract – the solar plexus is known as 'the abdominal brain'.
Position: Firm hollow, immediately below the hard ball, to the centre of the fleshy instep on the soles of the feet.

Everyone feels vulnerable from time to time!

The solar plexus, a network of sympathetic nerves, is directly linked to the abdominal organs and because it controls emotions, the digestive tract is immediately affected by nervousness and extreme anxiety e.g. 'butterflies in the stomach', diarrhoea etc.

Mood changes, instantly interpreted by the solar plexus, are physically manifested throughout the mind, body and soul. In Reflexology, the powerful solar plexus reflexes are used to calm deep distress, stop asthmatic attacks and soothe anxiety.

The right reflex reflects past emotional control, whilst the left solar plexus reflex mirrors present sentiments.

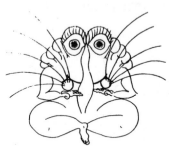

THE POSITION OF THE SOLAR PLEXUS
REFLEXES

CHARACTERISTICS OF THE
SOLAR PLEXUS REFLEX

- Solar plexus reflexes are naturally supple but firm hollows immediately below the hard balls on both feet.

Only when we are no longer afraid do we begin to enjoy life and live in gratitude!

THE EFFECT OF THE SUBCONSCIOUS MIND
ON THE SOLAR PLEXUS

Firm, vibrant hollow: Healthy and well-balanced, controlling all aspects of the self.

Swollen: Weighed down by heavy or unresolved emotions.

Sunken: Emotionally drained and feeling totally flat. Lack of emotional control.

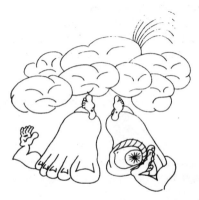

SUNKEN SOLAR PLEXUS:
DRAINED OF EMOTION

Wavy lines: Overcome by waves of emotion.
Lines emitting downwards:
　The number of lines indicates
　the number of activities that
　draw on the emotions
　hampering progress.

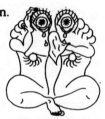

LINES FROM SOLAR PLEXUS:
EMOTIVE ACTIVITIES

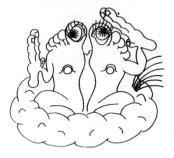

ARC OVER SOLAR PLEXUS:
PROTECTING THE EMOTIONS

Distinct line or arc over the
　top: Keeping someone at bay
　due to the emotional upheaval
　they cause.

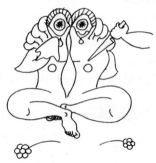

DAGGER MARKINGS:
FEELING STABBED TO THE CORE

Dagger-shaped marking:
　Feeling 'stabbed in the chest'
　and attacked causing
　emotional havoc.

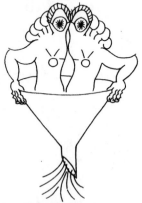

FUNNEL MARKINGS: DRAINED OF
EMOTIONS

Funnel-shaped lines from the
　base of the hollow: A feeling
　that 'the plug has been pulled
　out'. Deflated and flat from
　emotions draining away. When
　these lines are below the solar
　plexus on the right foot but
　above the solar plexus on the
　left foot, past emotions have
　been released and no longer
　drain the whole, whilst present
　emotions have been lifted onto
　a more manageable plane.

The Third Toe and its Related Parts, The Upper Half of the Instep Including the Liver, Stomach, Pancreatic, Spleen and Transverse Colon Reflexes

THE THIRD TOE - THE DOING TOE

Symbolises: Self-empowerment and instinctive survival.
Qualities: Appropriate responses and actions.
Element: Fire to provide the energy and enthusiasm to motivate activity.
Colour: Yellow.
Related to: The middle finger and upper instep.
Connection: The digestive system.
Direct reflexes: On the soles of the feet: Liver, gall-bladder, stomach, pancreas, spleen, transverse colon, adrenal glands, heart and solar plexus.
Indirect reflexes: On the top and the sides of the feet: Middle back, central spine and elbow.

Learn to love to do well and you will!

The fiery third toe motivates and fuels active thoughts and encourages them to be put into practice.

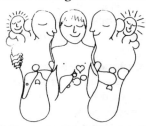

Mobile thoughts, mirrored onto the third toe, are influenced by basic emotions, feelings (the second toe) and intellectual knowledge (big toe).

The right third toe reflects past impressions of agile thoughts, whilst the left third toe displays present thoughts of endeavour.

THE THIRD TOE AND ITS RELATED PARTS IN THE UPPER INSTEP

CHARACTERISTICS OF THE THIRD TOE

- A straight, upstanding, flexible third toe is active, inventive and capable of tackling any task.
- The length of the third toe indicates potential for conscientious enthusiasm. The longer the toe, the greater the energy and drive.
- The shape and size of the pad on the third toe is related to the prospective amount of thought regarding activity.
- The neck of the third toe encourages the two-way expression of the cause and effect of actions.

PARTS RELATED TO THE THIRD TOE

Solar plexus: Feelings and emotions control activity. Too much or too little will determine the way in which things are done. When feeling good and in control, life is a breeze!

Heart: Unconditionally does things with love, by putting the 'heart and soul' into it! A happy heart finds things easier to do!

Stomach: Provides fuel and energy for activity. Breaks down life's events for absorption and development. 'Butterflies' in the stomach indicate anxiety and concern for future events.

Liver: Stores energy to fuel the whole. Provides drive, enthusiasm and get up and go. The seat of primitive emotions, such as anger, frustration etc., which has a destructive effect and saps the whole of energy.

Gall-bladder: Releases obstacles that otherwise hamper progress. If resentment is not released, bitterness builds up and is a deterrent to peaceful activity.

Spleen: Provides uniformity and guidelines for the way in which actions are performed. Stores current emotions which determine the manner in which activity is pursued. If too obsessive the balance is tipped.

Pancreas: Ability to absorb and appreciate the sweetness of life. Affects the energy level. Hypoglycaemia indicates lack of enthusiasm.

Adrenal glands: Provide force and super-human strength, particularly during life-threatening situations. Often 'burnt-out' due to imagined fear.

Middle back: Supports and backs all activity. Remorse, disappointment and guilt from failing to achieve or meet expectations is tucked into the small of the back, affecting future activities.

Elbow: Eases changes in directions. Resistance to activities may lead to the perception that it is necessary 'to elbow one's way through life'.

Transverse colon: Determines the amount of pressure required to do things successfully. Too much pressure from the self or others, due to never being satisfied with outstanding achievements, puts strain on the whole.

> *There are three kinds of people:*
> *those who make things happen;*
> *those who watch things happen;*
> *and those who wondered what happened!*

THE INFLUENCE OF THE SUBCONSCIOUS MIND ON THE THIRD TOE

Life is easy when we don't complicate and confuse it!

Flexible: Actively thinks through tasks. Capable of achieving anything the mind is set on. Energetic and inventive. Feels good about its activity and puts its 'heart and soul' into everything.

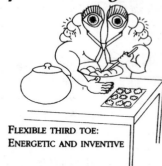

FLEXIBLE THIRD TOE: ENERGETIC AND INVENTIVE

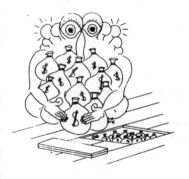

Rigid: Inflexible thoughts regarding the way in which activities are performed. Obstinate. Perfectionist or insecure with selfish, set ways.

RIGID THIRD TOE: DEFINITE IDEAS OF HOW TO DO THINGS

✳ *85*

Squashed: Limited and restricted from inventing, let alone activating own ideas. Feeling that the hands are tied. Children and the elderly are often prevented from doing things for themselves.

Bashed: Frustrated at not being able to put perceptions and thoughts into practice because considered insubordinate, inadequate or of no value. Obstacles block own ideas.

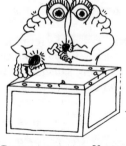

BASHED THIRD TOE: UNABLE TO PUT THOUGHTS INTO PRACTICE

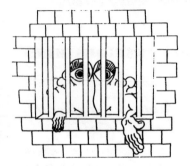

Crooked: Active thoughts altered to accommodate the ideas of others. Direction changed from own way of thinking.

CROOKED THIRD TOE: DOING TO PLEASE OTHERS

Stands back: Self-conscious and anxious of the opinion of others. Fears possible disgrace or rejection.

Reflexology footnotes

* THE FIERY ASPECT OF THE THIRD FINGER MOTIVATES AND INSPIRES CONFIDENCE.
* AN ITCHY THIRD TOE IS ITCHING TO GET ON AND DO THINGS WHILST FLAKING SKIN INDICATES AN IMPATIENT DESIRE TO BREAK AWAY TO DO ITS OWN THING!

THE UPPER HALF OF THE INSTEP

Symbolises: The manifestation of physical, emotional and spiritual control, achievements and basic survival.
Qualities: The appropriate response to all situations.
Element: Fire to fuel activity.
Colour: Yellow.
Related to: The third toe and middle finger.
Direct reflexes: On the soles of the feet: Liver, duodenum, stomach, spleen, pancreas, adrenal glands, transverse colon and solar plexus.
Indirect reflexes: On the top and sides of the feet: Middle back, central spine and elbow.

Act as if everything makes the difference!

The fiery aspect of the upper instep activates the thoughts of the third toe. It reflects:

* THE ABILITY TO COPE WITH CHALLENGES WITHOUT BEING DISCOURAGED AND DISILLUSIONED.
* THE CONFIDENCE AND KNOWLEDGE THAT EVERYTHING CARRIED OUT HAS BEEN EFFECTIVELY EXECUTED WITH REALISTIC EXPECTATIONS, AND IN THE INTERESTS OF ALL CONCERNED.
* THE CONTROL OF EMOTIONS TO AVOID INTERFERENCE AND HAVOC.

The right upper instep reveals past activity, whilst the left reflects present actions.

CHARACTERISTICS OF THE UPPER HALF OF THE INSTEP

* Upper insteps are naturally flesh-coloured, vibrant and blemish-free. They enjoy the immediacy of life, without feeling pressurised, and move on without being marked or held back by unresolved emotions.

It's not what we do, but how we do it!

THE INFLUENCE OF THE SUBCONSCIOUS MIND ON THE UPPER INSTEP

Vibrant and pliable: Puts ideas into action with confidence and enthusiasm. Totally in control.

Wrinkled: Exhausted from trying to implement own ideas or from meeting the demands of others.

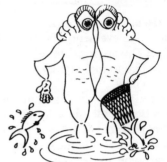

WRINKLED UPPER INSTEP:
DRAINED OF ENTHUSIASM!

Lines from solar plexus reflexes: The number of actions that are emotionally draining, or activities done with compassion and feeling.

Swollen adrenal reflexes: Extra resources required to deal with particularly demanding situations. A perceived need to safeguard the self or be continually on the defensive. Particularly evident on people with impaired sight.

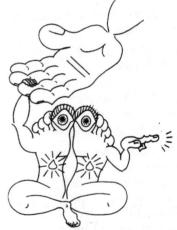

SWOLLEN ADRENAL REFLEXES:
EXTREME ANXIETY

Collapsed instep: Giving in to pressure and unrealistic expectations. Feeling totally unsupported in activities.

Burning instep: Inflamed about activities.

Itching instep: Itching to get on!

THE STOMACH REFLEXES

Symbolises: The physical adaptation of life-forces to fuel mind, body and soul.
Qualities: Ability to utilise life's experiences advantageously.
Element: Fire to provide energy and enthusiasm.
Colour: Yellow.
Position on the feet: Immediately below the hard balls of the feet on the inner, upper aspects of the fleshy insteps.

The work of the individual is the spark that moves mankind forward.

The stomach accepts or rejects food, as well as thoughts, ideas, perceptions and life's experiences that have been chewed over and swallowed.

Nutritious forces fuel thoughts that feed the mind. If palatable and digestible, food and life experiences are easily converted to facilitate absorption for the growth and development of mind, body and soul.

Stomach reflexes mirror the influence of feelings and emotions in this process and provide fuel for the thoughts of the third toe to be put into action.

The right stomach reflex reflects remnants of past experiences, that provide input and knowledge of how to deal with current situations, whilst the bulk of the stomach reflexes, on the left foot, relate to present/future situations. This is significant since the greatest anxiety arises from the fear of not coping with forthcoming events or present circumstances, such as writing an examination or starting a new job.

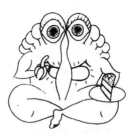

THE POSITION OF THE
STOMACH REFLEXES

CHARACTERISTICS OF THE STOMACH REFLEXES

- Stomach reflexes are naturally flesh-coloured, slightly raised, vibrant mounds.

THE EFFECT OF THE SUBCONSCIOUS MIND ON THE STOMACH REFLEXES

Swollen: Weighed down by the need to 'stomach' unpalatable circumstances. Overcome by the enormity of it all!

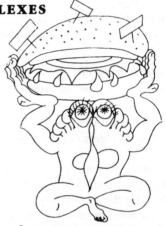

SWOLLEN STOMACH REFLEXES:
TOO MUCH TO STOMACH!

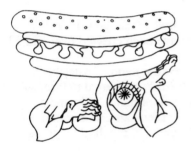

SUNKEN STOMACH REFLEXES:
EXHAUSTED FROM STOMACHING LIFE!

Sunken: Drained at all that is having to be stomached. Eating away at the self.

Lined: Compartmentalises certain aspects of life to be broken down step by step. Likes to deal with one thing at a time.

Faint, random lines: Fluttering anxiety and concern. Uneasy about having to deal with certain life experiences.

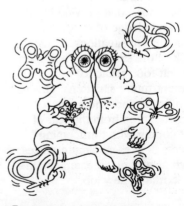

BUTTERFLIES IN THE STOMACH

Deep crevice between stomach and heart: Loving feelings kept separate from activities, to prevent heartache or to avoid getting too emotionally involved in activities, e.g. a nurse handling so many heart-rending situations.

'Butterflies' in the stomach are fine when they fly in formation!

THE LIVER REFLEXES

Symbolises: Abundant energy for creative activity.
Qualities: Balanced control of emotions for the fair distribution of essential life-forces.
Element: Fire to fuel activities with ongoing energy.
Colour: Yellow.
Position on the feet: A triangular-shaped mound, predominantly on the right fleshy instep, with a tip of the reflex at the top of the left inner fleshy instep.

Lack of energy arises from living an artificial, unfulfilling experience.

The liver contains vital primal emotions to ensure survival. It relentlessly provides an on-going supply of fiery energy to fuel all conscious and unconscious activities.

Constructive actions energise the whole, filling it with boundless enthusiasm, whereas destructive action drains mind, body and soul of vitality, leaving the whole deflated and exhausted.

Poisonous substances, including toxic thoughts and words, are rejected by the liver to maintain a state of homoeostasis.

The balance is upset when suppressed anger and frustration fester and erupt because personal belief systems and principles are perceived to be under attack or threatened.

The bulk of the liver reflex is on the right foot since only emotions that have been experienced can be stored.

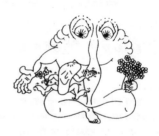

POSITION OF THE LIVER REFLEX

CHARACTERISTICS OF THE LIVER REFLEXES

- Healthy liver reflexes are vibrant, pliable and naturally rounded, indicating effective and efficient functioning.

With so much talent, what a pity to waste it!

THE EFFECT OF THE SUBCONSCIOUS MIND ON LIVER REFLEXES

Sunken: Drained of energy and vitality due to the destructive effect of stored, resentful emotions.

Bulging: Filled with anger and frustration. Extremely critical of others to justify own reactions.

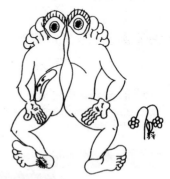

SUNKEN LIVER REFLEXES: DRAINED OF ENERGY AND VITALITY

BULGING LIVER REFLEXES: FILLED WITH ANGER AND FRUSTRATION

Criticism is the adult way of crying.

Reflexology footnotes

* LIVER REFLEXES SWELL CONSIDERABLY DURING DETOXIFICATION OR ON STRICT VEGANS.
* CONCENTRATE ON MASSAGING THE LIVER REFLEX FOR THE RELEASE OF SUPPRESSED EMOTIONS THAT HAVE BEEN STORED AND HAMPER PROGRESS.
* STROKE THE LIVER REFLEX WITH THE THIRD FINGER FOR THE RELEASE OF ENERGY TO FIRE THE WHOLE WITH CONSTRUCTIVE ENTHUSIASM.

THE PANCREATIC REFLEXES

Symbolises: The sweet and charming aspects of life.
Qualities: Control and understanding through experiencing the quality of life.
Element: Fire to inspire.
Colour: Yellow.
Position on the feet: Immediately above the 'waistline' of both feet, along the inner aspect of the fleshy insteps.

Mind, body and soul thrive on correct nourishment and sweetness of thought, word and deed.

The pancreas injects mind, body and soul with substances that sweeten thoughts, gratify emotions and inspire enjoyment of the nectar of life.

At the same time, it assists with the breakdown and release of life's toxic and emotional remnants which, otherwise, would create a bitter and putrid environment.

Pancreatic reflexes reflect the amount of love and joy being replenished, or the quantity required, to keep a balanced, agreeable state throughout.

The right pancreatic reflex mirrors past impressions of harmonious events, whilst the left pancreatic reflex reflects the amount of gratification derived from current experiences.

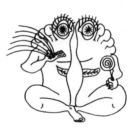

CHARACTERISTICS OF THE PANCREATIC REFLEXES

CHARACTERISTICS OF THE PANCREATIC REFLEXES

- Healthy pancreatic reflexes form a flesh-coloured, vibrant, tadpole-shaped mound that stretches across the inner halves of both fleshy insteps, just above the 'waistline'.

THE INFLUENCE OF THE SUBCONSCIOUS MIND ON THE PANCREATIC REFLEXES

Vibrant mounds: Break down old, wasted emotions to make space for the new, refreshing aspects of life, thereby creating sweet harmony throughout the whole.

Swollen: Overcome with emotion and unable to break down old feelings, which contaminate the present. Overwhelming need for energy and sweetness to provide a boost.

Flattened: Exhausted and drained from trying to stay in control. Deflated from the sweet aspects being drained out of the substance of life.

THE SPLEEN REFLEX

Symbolises: Personal pursuits and physical precision.
Qualities: Appropriate actions and responses.
Element: Fire.
Colour: Yellow.
Position on the feet: A small fleshy circular mound, on the outer, upper aspect of the fleshy instep on the left foot only.

Our greatest obsession should be to enjoy life!

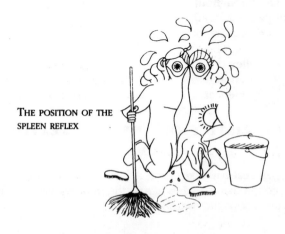

THE POSITION OF THE
SPLEEN REFLEX

The spleen reflex reflects the degree of precision required for the creative accomplishment of activities.

Current emotions, stored in this bodily part, balance obsessional behaviour that would otherwise 'tip the balance'.

CHARACTERISTICS OF THE SPLEEN REFLEX

- The spleen reflex is a naturally rounded, pliable, flesh-coloured mound on the **left foot** only.

THE EFFECT OF THE SUBCONSCIOUS MIND ON THE SPLEEN REFLEX

Vibrant: Enthusiastically guides activities.
Swollen: Inclined to obsessive behaviour. Over-concerned and particular about the way in which things are done. Over-sensitive.

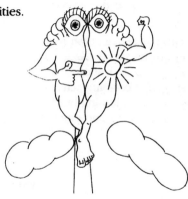

SWOLLEN SPLEEN REFLEX: OBSESSIONAL!

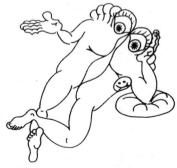

FLATTENED SPLEEN REFLEX:
TOO EASY-GOING!

Flattened: Little concern for the manner in which activities are pursued. Too easy-going.

Reflexology footnote

∗ AN ENLARGED SPLENIC REFLEX DURING A MALARIAL ATTACK REFLECTS A CHARACTERISTIC OBSESSIONAL STREAK COMMON AMONGST MALARIAL SUFFERERS, WHO TEND TO BE NEUROTIC ABOUT TAKING ANTI-MALARIAL TABLETS, AND YET STILL MANIFEST THE DIS-EASE.

THE TRANSVERSE COLON REFLEXES

Symbolises: The ability to let go.
Qualities: Eases the flow of life.
Element: Fire and water.
Colour: Yellow and orange.
Position on feet: Across the 'waistline' of both feet, rising slightly on the far aspect of the left foot.

No one person is perfect in a world of individuals!

The transverse colon reflexes mirror balanced relationships and communications that make space for ongoing activity to occur, by releasing burdensome, wasteful tasks and emotions.

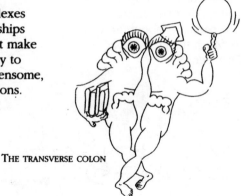

THE TRANSVERSE COLON

CHARACTERISTICS OF THE TRANSVERSE COLON REFLEXES

- The colon reflexes should be naturally flat, smooth, pink and pliable.

THE EFFECT OF THE SUBCONSCIOUS MIND ON THE TRANSVERSE COLON REFLEXES

Vibrant and viable: Able to let go and move on with ease.
Swollen: Unrealistically high expectations of the self or others.

Usually great achievers and perfectionists always wanting to do better than their best!

Sunken: Drained of energy and enthusiasm due to too much pressure.

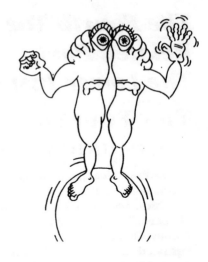

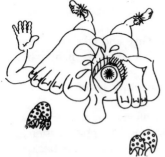

SWOLLEN TRANSVERSE COLON:
UNREALISTICALLY HIGH EXPECTATIONS

SUNKEN TRANSVERSE COLON:
GIVEN IN UNDER PRESSURE

Flattened: Disappointment at not being able to achieve high expectations.

Greater regret is experienced for those things not done, than for those that have been done!

The Fourth Toe and the Related Part, The Lower Instep

THE FOURTH TOE – THE COMMUNICATING TOE

Symbolises: Pleasurable thoughts that enhance relationships and communication.

Qualities: Accommodating and adaptable. Give and take with ease.

Element: Water, the medium of transport that connects many parts.

Colour: Orange.

Connection: Circulatory, lymphatic and excretory systems.

Related to: Ring finger and lower instep.

Direct reflexes: On the soles of the feet: Small intestines, large colon, kidneys, Fallopian tubes, uterus, circulatory and lymphatic systems.

Indirect reflexes: On the tops and sides of the feet: Lower back, lower arms and calves.

The watery aspect of the fourth toe allows for the lively exchange of thoughts and life-forces and, through the smooth flow of communication, enhances relationships and emotional pleasure.

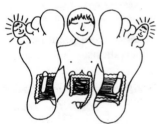

THE FOURTH TOE AND RELATED AREAS

The right fourth toe reflects past impressions of thoughts regarding communication and relationships, whereas the left fourth toe reflects those of the present.

CHARACTERISTICS OF THE FOURTH TOE

- A straight, upstanding, flexible fourth toe is naturally affectionate, accommodating, humble and compassionate.
- The natural length of the fourth toe indicates potential confidence to express ideas regarding relationships and communication.

- The size and shape of the pad of the fourth toe indicate the amount of affection available and the potential to communicate. It is particularly large on those who utilise their skills, e.g. teachers, actors, broadcasters, etc.
- The neck of the fourth toe encourages the free exchange of life-forces.

AREAS RELATED TO THE FOURTH TOE

Small intestines: Absorb beneficial substances and feelings for growth and development, and release those without value, thereby enhancing communication and relationships.

Large colon: Reduces pressure by working through things to prevent being 'bogged down' by wasted emotions.

Kidneys: Process and discard all that is not required to avoid build-up of wasted emotions. Retain beneficial substances for effectual distribution.

Fallopian tubes: The ovum and the sperm meet and may fertilise in the tube, allowing a new relationship to grow and develop.

Uterus: Nourishes new life and provides space for growth and expansion. Menstruation changes the environment, on a monthly basis, for any new developments.

Circulatory system: Circulates love, vitality and joy throughout to nourish the whole and encourage good relationships. The blood continually provides the brain with information regarding the state of bodily parts. If two-way communication is agreeable a healthy relationship is maintained.

Lymphatic system: The sewerage system that eliminates anything that threatens gratifying relationships or communications. Defends the whole for a harmonious environment.

Lower back: Provides support and backs all forms of life. The basis upon which good communication and relationships can develop.

Lower arms: The arms open to embrace and extend to shake hands, sealing agreements and enhancing relationships.

Reproductive organs: Sexual intimacy is the highest form of physical communication between two people.

People are lonely because they build walls
instead of bridges.

THE INFLUENCE OF THE SUBCONSCIOUS MIND ON THE FOURTH TOE

To give is to receive.

Flexible: Exchanges ideas with ease and confidence and is accommodating. Open and honest in dealings with others.

FLEXIBLE FOURTH TOE: HONEST AND ACCOMMODATING

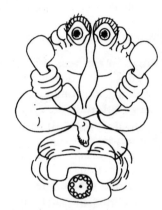

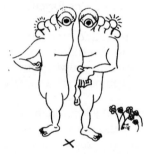

RIGID FOURTH TOE: HIGHLY PRINCIPLED!

Rigid: Strongly principled with firm belief systems. Very definite ideas on how to communicate and on the nature of relationships.

Squashed: Restricted in display of affection and inhibited about sharing ideas and perceptions.

SQUASHED FOURTH TOE: INHIBITED IN DISPLAY OF EMOTIONS

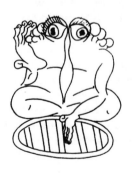

Believe in the self.

Bent: Bends to please others. Feels dominated, distrustful and defensive. Not standing up to own ideas, or having difficulty in communicating personal thoughts for fear of ridicule.

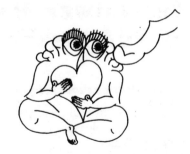

BENT FOURTH TOE: BENDING TO PLEASE OTHERS

Crooked: Not straight in dealings. Goes 'around the houses' to do things. Pleasing others rather than following own ideas.

Turns in: Shy and lacks confidence to face the world openly and express the self.

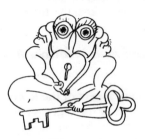

SHY FOURTH TOE: UNABLE TO FACE THE WORLD!

Communicate freely with love, joy and enthusiasm.

Reflexology footnote

✱ THE RING FINGER FILLS THE WHOLE WITH PLEASURABLE VIBRANCY AND IS USED IN REFLEXOLOGY FOR INNER HARMONY.

THE LOWER HALF
OF THE INSTEP

Communications and relationships

Symbolises: Physical relationships and communication.
Qualities: The pleasure and enjoyment of life.
Element: Water.
Colour: Orange.
Related to: Fourth toe and ring finger.
Direct reflexes: On the soles of the feet: Small intestine, large colon, kidneys, ureters, uterus, Fallopian tubes, ovaries.
Indirect reflexes: On the tops and sides of the feet: Lower back, bladder, lower arms and lower legs.

Every new relationship is an opportunity to heal the past.

The watery aspect of the lower instep connects it directly to the bottom part of the digestive tract, as well as the kidneys, the circulatory and lymphatic systems.

It mirrors the natural ability of mind, body and soul to sift through life's experiences so that beneficial data can be constructively utilised, whilst unnecessary, wasteful burdens can be released to make space for beneficial personal development and progress.

It displays the manner in which the thoughts, ideas and concepts of the fourth toe are put into practice.

Tension and anxiety restrict the flow of natural life-forces and prevent the effective distribution and uptake of essential life-forces and release of toxic substances.

The lower instep contains the female reproductive glands and organ reflexes. The union of two energies, the sperm and the ova, creates new life-forces, extending the relationship between two people.

The right lower half of the fleshy instep reflects impressions of past relationships, whilst the left lower instep reflects present communication and liaisons.

Keep the lines of communication open by choosing words carefully and really listening to what others say.

CHARACTERISTICS OF THE LOWER HALF OF THE INSTEP

- The lower instep is naturally smooth, vibrant and flesh-coloured.

THE EFFECT OF THE SUBCONSCIOUS MIND ON THE LOWER HALF OF INSTEP

Lack of involvement leads to loneliness and despair!

Vibrant and pliable: Sifts through life's experiences with ease and confidence, enhancing communication and relationships.

Transverse ripples: So much going on. Wading through life. Up and down. Heavy going. Not sure what to absorb and what to dismiss. Pronounced ripples indicate being stuck in a rut.

RIPPLED INSTEP: 'STUCK IN A RUT'

Scattered lines: Confusion. Unable to absorb all that is happening. No firm direction.

Diagonally crossed lines: Feels entrapped and caught in a net hampering communications and relationships, creating conflict.

Sunken and pale: Giving up trying to be understood, or exhausted from a draining or demanding relationship.

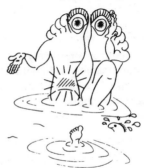

SUNKEN, PALE INSTEP: TOTALLY DRAINED OF ENERGY

Don't wait around for others to make you happy - happiness comes from within!

Bulging: Weighed down from having to absorb life's events. On women, it may indicate pregnancy.

Stain over uterine reflex on left foot: Trying to fall pregnant, or perceived sexual abuse.

White, sunken uterine reflex: Possible miscarriage or disillusionment with femineity.

Swollen: Feeling bloated and resisting the flow. Disinterested and disenchanted with life. If pregnant, the position and shape of the baby is reflected onto the bottom of the instep as soon as the uterus expands noticeably.

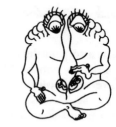

PREGNANT REFLEX: THE GIFT OF LIFE

Accommodate the self and others!

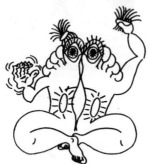

Swollen kidney reflexes: Humiliated, frustrated, disappointed and depressed. Tends to be dissatisfied with everything and everyone.

SWOLLEN KIDNEY REFLEXES: DISILLUSIONED AND DEPRESSED

Collapsed: Feeling completely 'flat' and unsupported in a relationship. Babies and children are naturally flat-footed until they have the inner strength to support themselves rather than be dependent on others.

The Little Toe and its Related Part, The Heels

THE LITTLE TOE - THE MOBILE TOE

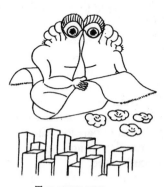

THE LITTLE TOE:
MOBILITY OF THOUGHT

Symbolises: Freedom and expansion of thought for the security to believe in personal concepts.

Qualities: Mental agility and mobility.

Element: Earth provides a solid basis from which to grow, develop and progress.

Colour: Red – the lowest colour vibration.

Connection: Skeletal system.

Related to: The little finger and the heels.

Direct reflexes: On the soles of the feet: Pelvic area, feet, reproductive glands and organs.

Indirect reflexes: On the tops of the feet: Buttocks, anus, rectum, bladder, lower back, feet, hands, reproductive glands and organs.

A wise man refuses to be confined and limited to the restrictions of the physical world and uses the expansive mind to achieve ultimate fulfilment!

The earth element of the little toe keeps it firmly on the ground, giving it security, freedom and space to grow and develop.

Related and influenced by family relationships, its characteristics are moulded according to the amount of dependence, independence and interdependence.

Expansive, mobile thoughts, frequently inhibited by family and social belief systems, become restricted, leading to resentment and frustration.

Personal identity is inevitably lost in the falsehood and charade of life, perceived to be necessary to meet other's expectations. Hence, most little toes are squashed or insignificant-looking.

Self-imposed restrictions close the mind to greater ideas, thereby limiting individual scope and potential.

Thinking, imprisoned and inhibited by greed and a desire for physical possessions, is confined by the belief that the only security lies in the material world of accumulated wealth. This misguided perception hinders personal expansion into the world of truth and anchors the little toe through fear and insecurity.

The greater the insecurity, the greater the limitation and impact on the little toe. With security comes expansiveness of thought, freeing the little toe and giving it the space to express its true personality.

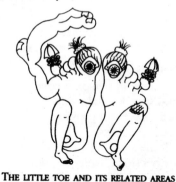

The right little toe reflects past impressions of thoughts regarding mobility and inner security, whilst the left little toe reflects those in the present.

THE LITTLE TOE AND ITS RELATED AREAS

We find comfort amongst those who agree with us, but growth amongst those who don't!

CHARACTERISTICS OF THE LITTLE TOE

- A mobile, upstanding little toe nurtures and cares for life. Its security provides a solid foundation for progress, flexibility and independence.

- The natural length of the little toe indicates potential space for freedom and mobility of thought.
- The size and shape of the pad on the little toe demonstrates potential access to unrestricted thoughts.
- The neck of the little toe allows for the two-way exchange of thoughts and activity for security, growth, development and the confidence to move ahead.

*Stagnation is the price of tyranny;
prosperity is the reward of freedom!*

PARTS RELATED TO THE LITTLE TOE

Pelvis: The bony structure provides support and the thrust to progress ahead.

Feet: The flexibility and adaptability of the feet are determined by the amount of enthusiasm to expand and explore life to the full.

Hands: If secure, life's experiences are handled and moulded with ease.

Reproductive glands: Provide on-going energy for the expansion of life.

Reproductive organs: In women, enlarges to accommodate the development of new life.

Buttocks: The pride and power to move ahead with confidence.

Rectum and anus: The ability to release the old for new experiences to be encountered.

Bladder: Stores excessive substances for release and expulsion, creating space for progress.

Lower back: Supports and provides a solid foundation from which the whole can expand, grow and develop.

THE EFFECT OF THE SUBCONSCIOUS MIND ON THE LITTLE TOE

Simply be yourself!

Flexible: Sympathetic, nurturing, supportive, patient, dependable and considerate. Changes and adapts to accommodate life's adventures.

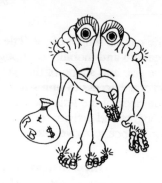

Rigid: Cautious, unenterprising and deliberate. Set beliefs, obstructive and anchored to the materialistic world. Extremely insecure.

RIGID LITTLE TOE: ANCHORED TO THE PHYSICAL WORLD!

Stands alone: Eager to cover new ground and break away. Ready to move on.

Ridge of hard skin: Impregnable but concerned. Protection from seeing the greed, scepticism or pessimism of modern society. Two ways of thinking; one is exposed and the other kept to the self.

Squashed: No time or space to create a firm foundation. Reluctant to take on further 'responsibilities', particularly within the family. Movement and progress inhibited. Apprehensive from breaking away from the tried and tested.

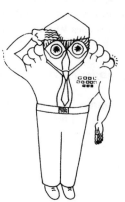

SQUASHED LITTLE TOE: INHIBITED AND INSECURE

Dented: Feeling vulnerable because mobility and security are knocked or threatened.

Time is:
Too slow for those who wait,
Too swift for those who fear,
Too long for those who grieve,
Too short for those who rejoice,
But for those who show love,
Time is eternity.

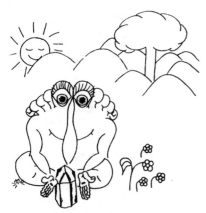

Turns in: Back turned on the senseless aspects of today's society. To keep the peace, its mobile, often ethereal, thoughts are modified. Common on 'new age' thinkers.

ETHEREAL LITTLE TOE: PREFERS PEACEFUL, LOVING THOUGHTS

Twisted: Turns away because discontent with restrictions. Anxious and frustrated at not being able to move ahead with ease.

Bent: Troubled and overburdened by physical possessions or lack of them. Easily influenced. Bends to please others. Conceals fear and anxiety.

BENT, ANXIOUS LITTLE TOE: GIVES IN TO SOCIAL AND FAMILY PRESSURES

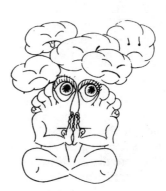

Reflexology footnotes

✳ MOVEMENT OF THE LITTLE TOE DURING A REFLEXOLOGY TREATMENT INDICATES A SHIFT IN CONSCIOUSNESS AND READINESS TO THINK MORE EXPANSIVELY, OPENING THE MIND TO NEW EXPERIENCES BY BREAKING TIES WITH THE PAST.

✳ THE LITTLE FINGER, WITH ITS GROUNDING EFFECT, BRINGS THOSE WITH THEIR HEADS IN THE CLOUDS DOWN TO EARTH!

THE HEELS

Symbolises: Freedom and space.
Qualities: Mobility and security for growth, movement and
  development.
Element: Earth – a firm base from which to grow and develop.
Colour: Red.
Related to: The little toe, little finger and skeletal system.
Direct reflexes: Pelvis, hips, lower limbs, feet, hands, reproductive
  organs and glands.
Indirect reflexes: Buttocks, lower back, anus, rectum, bladder,
  reproductive glands and organs.

It's impossible to move forwards backwards!

The earthly heels provide a secure base for personal growth and
development. The hip, lower limb and feet reflexes, mirrored onto
the heels, physically manifest and mobilise the thoughts, ideas and
perceptions of the little toe.

The influence of masculinity and femininity on individual progress
is displayed through the reproductive reflexes, which project their
energy in an attempt to reproduce mankind.

Male reproductive glands and organs, reflected onto heels and
ankles, indicate the need for the firm basis essential for procreation.

With feet securely grounded, legs can confidently step ahead and
willingly explore the expansiveness of life's mysteries. Those with a
thirst for life, particularly children, are constantly on the go, and
eagerly seek new adventures for growth and development. Others,
burdened with emotions and responsibilities, drag their feet
begrudgingly down life's path.

The right heel reflects impressions of past mobility and stability,
whilst the left heel reflects present impressions.

CHARACTERISTICS OF THE HEEL

• A balanced heel is a pliable, pink, unblemished mound.

Time is precious – once spent, it cannot be refunded!

THE MEANINGS OF THE VARIOUS SECTIONS OF THE HEEL

Inner edge: Intuitively secure with ideas and thoughts, so can move ahead and progress with ease.

Between inner edge and centre: Feeling secure and emotionally uninhibited.

Centre: Happy with activities, so able to grow and expand without constraint.

Between outer edge and centre: Confident that communications and relationships enhance development.

Outer edge: Untroubled and able to adapt to life's ups and downs with ease. A solid foundation.

Unconditional love has always met, and will always meet, every human need!

THE EFFECTS OF THE SUBCONSCIOUS MIND ON THE HEEL

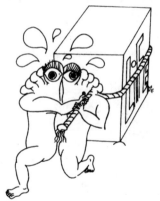

Vibrant: Secure and well-heeled. Covers new ground with confidence and ease.

Heavy: Overburdened and 'down at heel'. Finds life heavy going, and drags its way through life.

HEAVY HEEL: DRAGGING ITS WAY THROUGH LIFE

The greatest risk in life is to risk nothing!

Narrow: Treads carefully so as not to disturb or attract attention. Prefers not to be obvious. Devious movements arise from need to break away.

Swollen: Lacks energy or
enthusiasm to move on.
Perceives a bleak future.
Bogged down and lifeless.

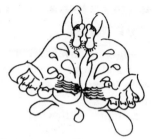

SWOLLEN HEELS: WEIGHED DOWN AND
DISILLUSIONED

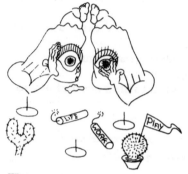

WRINKLED HEELS: PERCEIVED OBSTACLES!

Wrinkled: Obstacles anticipated
en route. Worried and
concerned about the journey
ahead. Anxious about security.
Would like to 'turn on the
heels'.

Cold: Lacks the confidence and enthusiasm to move ahead.
Intentions are good, but gets 'cold feet' at the last moment!

Only the person who takes risks is entirely free!

Burning: Inflamed at present
situation or has a 'burning
desire' to move on. Needs to
'cool the heels'.

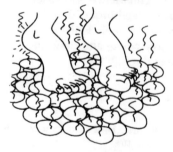

BURNING HEELS: CONSUMING AMBITION!

Bruised: 'Kicking the heels' and anxious to move on. Hurtful
situations perceived along the way. Movements 'knocked'.

Painful: 'Growing pains' due to personal development temporarily
being a painful experience. Life is perceivably 'a pain in the
buttocks', or progress and matters concerned with sexuality are
considered a pain.

Spongy: Indecisive and giving in.
Congested: Difficulty in moving ahead. Fearful and overwhelmed.
Rippled: 'Stuck in a rut' from the repetitive monotony of life.
Broad: A solid foundation.

Security is a state of mind!

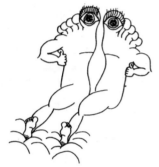

Hardened: 'Digging in' and refusing to budge! Reluctant to move on due to deep insecurity or determination to move ahead despite the odds. Unpenetrable.

HARDENED HEELS: DIGGING THE HEELS IN!

Spur: An anchor that inhibits progress. Deep hurt at being restrained. Needs to spurt ahead but reluctant to take the plunge.
Callous around edge: Protects gender, security or decisions from aggravating pressure to step ahead. In some females, the extra protection arises from a subconscious fear of falling pregnant!
Tyre around edge: Extra padding for increased security and to protect personal power. A more solid foundation. Reinforces defence, particularly of the gender.

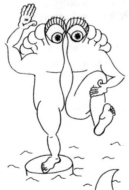

TYRE AROUND OUTER HEEL: EXTRA PROTECTION!

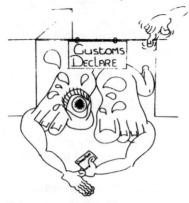

FLAKING HEEL: IRRITATED AT HAVING TO JUSTIFY MOVEMENTS!

Flaking skin over hard skin: Irritated at having to protect and justify movements.

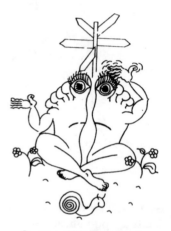

CRACKED HEEL: INDECISIVE!

Cracked: Security cracking up. Divided as to the way in which to proceed, due to inner turmoil and conflicting views. Pulled in many directions.

Shiny: Worn out from the friction, conflict and resistance encountered.

Festering blisters: Suppressed anger and frustration at encountered friction that threatens security, movement or sexuality. Simmering emotions now surface.

Extra bone at back of ankle: Perceived obstructions and obstacles to gender, security or mobility. Resistance to moving ahead or feeling held back.

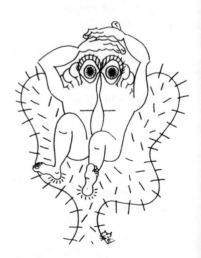

SHINY HEEL: CONSTANT FRICTION!

Line cutting off uterus: Moving ahead despite being a female in a male-dominant society or resentful at being cut off for being a female.

Black marks: Deep hurts from emotional or physical restrictions. Trying to move ahead in a prejudiced society.

BLACKENED HEEL: HAMPERED, HURTFUL PROGRESS

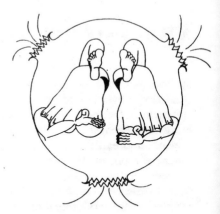

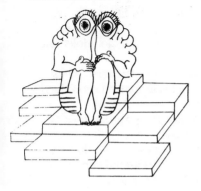

Stepped: Moves a step at a time. Cautious and insecure.

STEPPED HEEL: MOVES STEP BY STEP!

Every experience, 'good' and 'bad',
is an opportunity for growth and development.

REFLEXOLOGY FOOTNOTE

* THE HIGH INCIDENCE OF HEEL DISORDERS ARISES FROM GENERAL APATHY DUE TO INSECURITY WORLDWIDE AND FROM BEING TRAPPED IN A MATERIALISTIC, MONEY-ORIENTATED SOCIETY. REFLEXOLOGY RELEASES MIND, BODY AND SOUL FROM THIS IMPRISONMENT, ALLOWING EXPANSION AND DEVELOPMENT OF THE WHOLE.

The Top of the Feet, the Outer Edges of the Feet, the Instep

THE TOP OF THE FEET

Symbolises: Reinforced inner strength and support.
Qualities: Physical and emotional backing to security, relationships, activities, feelings, expressions and ideas.
Elements: From the tip of the toes to the ankles: Ether, air, fire, water and earth.
Colours: From the tip of the toes to the ankles: Indigo, violet, blue, green, yellow, orange and red.
Direct reflexes: On the top of the feet: Back of the head, neck, spine, lungs, abdominal organs, buttocks, limbs and reproductive organs.
Indirect reflexes: On the soles of the feet: Face, throat, breasts, shoulders, chest, abdominal organs, pelvis.

The bony, sinewy, muscular characteristics of the top of the foot provide a firm backing, reinforced strength and added support to carry the body, mind and soul through life's experiences.

The top of the feet reflect thoughts, emotions and activities that are perceived to be going on 'behind one's back' during particularly sensitive and vulnerable phases, or feelings that a back is turned, indicating abandonment and running away to avoid facing an issue. Also, that all is put behind us.

The top of the right foot reflects past impressions, and the top of the left foot those of the present.

CHARACTERISTICS OF THE TOP OF THE FEET

* The top of the foot is naturally flexible, strong and vibrant.

THE MEANINGS OF THE VARIOUS PARTS OF THE TOP OF THE FEET

To pinpoint the exact meaning of a marking, colouring or impression on the top of the foot, consult the following:

FROM THE TIPS OF THE TOES TO THE HEELS

Tops of toes: Support and endorses ideas.

Toe necks: Assist the two-way exchange of life's expressions.

Back of balls of feet: Provides emotional security and protection from being stabbed in the back.

Back of upper instep: Endorses actions and activities.

Back of lower instep: Assists communications and strengthens relationships.

Ankle: Adapts to life's ups and downs to provide a firm support and foundation for security, mobility and expansion.

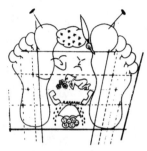

THE MEANING OF REFLEXES
ON TOP OF THE FOOT

FROM THE BIG TOE TO THE LITTLE TOE

Big toe: Substantiates and backs thoughts and actions of the intellect and intuitive mind.

Second toe: Helps thoughts of self-esteem and carries love in the heart.

Third toe: Assists ideas regarding activities and helps to put them into practice.

Fourth toe: Endorses ideas regarding communication and relationships and gives them the strength to become a reality.

Little toe: Favours expansive ideas and provides security for mobility and progress.

THE EFFECT OF THE SUBCONSCIOUS MIND ON THE TOP OF THE FEET

Tops of the feet – vibrant and strong: Supports and backs all life's experiences with enthusiasm and understanding.

Tops of toes – corns:

Above the toe joint: Protect ideas from being stamped and trampled upon.

Below the toe joint: Protect the expression of thoughts and perceptions.

On the sides of the toes: 'Turning a deaf ear' to protect the self from hearing emotionally disturbing aspects.

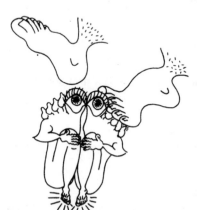

CORNS ON TOP OF FOOT:
GUARDING OWN IDEAS

Top of toe – misshapen: Direction of thought changed to accommodate another's belief system. Difficulty in following own dreams and ideas.

Top of foot – bunions: Rigidity either due to a strict upbringing or to strict self-discipline. Inflexibility gives the impression of bigotry. Wishes to break free of heavy emotions and feelings but is tied down by them.

Top of foot – prominent ligaments: Provide a strong 'back-up' to support ideas which need an iron rod to back them up. Pulling up own ideas in order to believe in them. Straining at the bit and rearing to get ahead. Feeling held back!

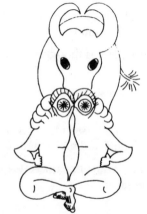

PROMINANT LIGAMENTS: WANTING
TO BREAK AWAY!

Top of foot – burning: Furious at all that is going on behind one's back.

Top of feet – protruding bone: Resistance to pressure to move ahead, especially when feeling driven and expected to meet endless demands. Feeling that the 'back is against the wall' and feeling hard pressed. Pushing the self.

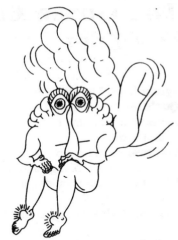

PROMINENT BONE: FEELING PRESSURISED!

Top of foot – red: Angry at having had the back 'put up' or at feeling that 'the back is against the wall'.

Top of foot – hairy: Protection from being ultra-sensitive about everything that is 'going on behind one's back'.

Top of foot – swollen: Weighed down by the burdens in life. Filled with unshed tears.

Top of foot – collapsed: Given in from having been over-burdened, breaking the back and bending over backwards. Back broken from having put everything into life.

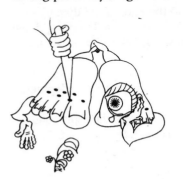

Top of foot – black marks or freckles: Feeling 'stabbed in the back'. Deeply hurt by all that is going on behind one's back.

Top of foot – wrinkled: Tired, worried or concerned by all that is going on 'behind one's back'.

BLACK MARKS OR FRECKLES: STABBED IN THE BACK!

Top of foot – strong imprint over hand reflex: Wishing to leave own mark or identity, otherwise at 'the beck and call of others'.

Top of foot – itchy hand reflexes: Impatient and wanting to mould own reality.

THE OUTER EDGES OF THE FEET

Symbolises: The ability to embrace and move ahead with ease.
Qualities: Freedom and mobility.
Elements: From the tips of the toes to the heels: ether, air, fire, water and earth.
Colours: From the tips of the toes to the heels: indigo, violet, blue, green, yellow, orange and red.
Direct reflexes: Shoulder, arm, elbow, knee, buttocks and side of body.
Indirect reflexes: All internal organs.

Act now for there is no time like the present!

The outer edges of the feet contribute balanced contours for security, mobility, growth and development of mind, body and soul. Limbs, free of fear and anxiety, explore and embrace life's potential with natural enthusiasm and ease. Feet move ahead into the unknown, whilst hands handle life's energies to create and mould a fulfilling reality. Flexible ankles and wrists spontaneously accommodate and cope with the variations of life's ups and downs. Limbs snap and break if pressurised into succumbing to the ego, rather than trusting the natural life forces. Hip reflexes, on the outer ankle bones, donate the major thrust in moving ahead, whilst buttock reflexes, on the outer heels, supply power to move.

Expressions, such as 'jumping for joy', ' walking with a spring in the step', 'dragging the feet' and so on, mirror the soul's adeptness, influencing the mobility of the soles.

Past impressions of security and progress mark the right outer foot, whilst those of the present rebound onto the left outer foot.

The only thing that is certain is that nothing is certain!

CHARACTERISTICS OF THE OUTER EDGES OF THE FOOT

- The outer edges of the feet are naturally firm but flexible, with an accommodating outline and slight undulations over the shoulder and elbow reflexes.

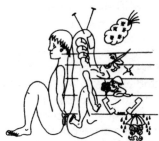

THE OUTER FOOT

THE MEANINGS OF THE OUTER FOOT REFLEXES

Little toe: Confidence and security with own ideas and thoughts.
Shoulder: Strength to shoulder and convey life's experiences.
Knee: The courage and faith to change direction and enjoy new experiences.
Upper arm: Accommodates and encourages the exchange of unconditional love.
Elbow: Adapts to changes in direction and innately controls creative activities.
Upper leg: Bolsters the whole along the path of life.
Lower arm: Opens to welcome, limit or reject the enormity of life. Accepts the self and others.
Feet: Established roots for stability, growth and development.
Hands: Handle and mould life's energies.
Buttocks: The power behind movement.
Hips: The thrust and enthusiasm to move ahead.

Experience is an effective teacher,
for wisdom comes through experience!

THE EFFECTS OF THE SUBCONSCIOUS MIND ON THE OUTER EDGES OF THE FOOT

Vibrant: Well supported and all-embracing. Adapts spontaneously and enthusiastically to changes.

Prominent shoulder joint reflex: Resists shouldering certain responsibilities or perceives the need to 'shove' a way through life.

Protruding upper arm reflexes: Straining to break free and escape from unresolved emotions and feelings. Requires space to embrace life more openly.

Rigid upper arm reflexes: Arms pinned to the sides. Keeps life and others at arm's length to avoid familiarity. Emotions kept close to the chest, feeling rebellious or 'up in arms'.

Sunken: Giving in to pressures and feeling that the 'stuffing has been knocked out'.

Swollen knee reflex: 'Knee deep' in emotion.

Prominent knee reflex: Inflexible and stubborn. Resists change, fearing ridicule or being considered weak-kneed or out of control.

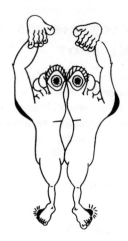

PROMINENT SHOULDER REFLEX: SHOULDERING WAY THROUGH LIFE!

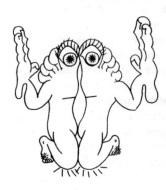

SWOLLEN KNEE REFLEX: KNEE DEEP IN EMOTION!

Prominent elbow reflex: Elbows way through life or reluctant to change direction. Needs to be in control. 'Up to the elbows' or 'no elbow room'.

PROMINENT ELBOW REFLEX: SHOVES WAY THROUGH LIFE!

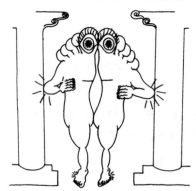

Swollen hand reflexes: Losing grip on life and feeling that everything is slipping through the fingers. Hands tied creating difficulty in handling life's events. Feeling 'all thumbs' or resentful at being under another's thumb.

Puffy hand reflex: Overwhelming pressure. Expectations out of reach or no longer at the finger tips.

Tense hand reflex: Tight-fisted. Not able to stretch out and handle the details of life.

Bluish swollen hand reflex: Hurt from continual resistance to natural creativity. Upset that not able to deal with situations.

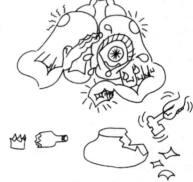

BRUISED HAND REFLEX: DIFFICULTY IN HANDLING LIFE!

Red hand reflexes: Angry and frustrated at having 'fingers burnt' or being 'twisted around someone else's fingers'.

Swollen outer ankle: Perceives a bleak future. Dissatisfaction with life in general. Fearful of stepping ahead. Seems to be little or no pleasure in life.

Outer heels – blue/black buttock reflex: Injured pride. Personal power under attack.

Swollen heels: Bogged down and powerless.

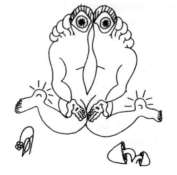

SWOLLEN HEELS: BOGGED DOWN AND POWERLESS!

All restrictions are self-imposed!

THE INSTEP

Symbolises: The backbone of life.
Qualities: Reliable strength and flexibility.
Elements: From the tip of the toes to the ankles: ether, air, fire, water and earth.
Colours: From the tip of the toes to the ankles: indigo, violet, blue, green, yellow, orange and red.
Direct reflexes: Midbrain, spinal cord, vertebrae, throat, oesophagus, heart, solar plexus, lungs, liver, pancreas, stomach, small intestine, colon, rectum, anus, bladder, urethra, sexual organs and sexual glands.

True support comes from within!

The bony ridge of the instep forms the backbone of the foot and reflects the spine. It strengthens mind, body and soul to allow the river of life to flow strongly and freely throughout.

All internal organs in the centre of the body are reflected onto the fleshy instep and mirror the ability to waltz through life, responding appropriately for personal growth and development.

The right instep reflects past support and encouragement, whilst the left mirrors impressions in the present.

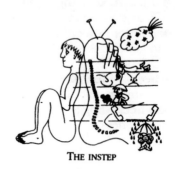

THE INSTEP

CHARACTERISTICS OF THE INSTEP

• The naturally strong and supple instep competently supports and accommodates the whole.

THE INSTEP AND RELATED SPINAL REFLEXES

Midbrain reflexes: Support and enforce perceptions.

Spinal cord reflexes: Confidently spreads ideas throughout the whole, making sure that the appropriate part of the body effectively activates them.

Neck reflexes: Flexibility to see every point of view. Scan the horizon for further ideas to back or expand present perceptions.

Upper back reflexes: Emotional backing and space for self-recognition.

Upper middle back reflexes: Actively support all actions and encourage appropriate responses.

Lower middle back reflexes: Fair distribution of life-forces to enhance communication and relationships.

Lower back reflexes: Foundation and base from which to grow and develop.

THE EFFECT OF THE SUBCONSCIOUS MIND ON THE BONY RIDGE OF THE INSTEP

Vibrant and supple: Firmly supports and provides inner strength to cope with ease.

A FIRM SUPPORT: COPES WITH EASE!

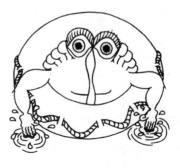

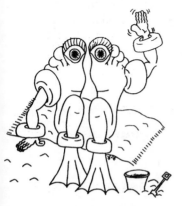

HIGH INSTEP: EXTRA SUPPORT

High instep: Draws extra strength from inner resources to support the self, especially during particularly demanding situations. Common on those who have had to support themselves from an early age, the bereaved or divorced parents who single-handedly support and nurture the family.

Flat instep: No backbone. Feeling unsupported and insecure. Heavily reliant upon the support of others. Babies and young children have naturally flat feet until they learn to support themselves.

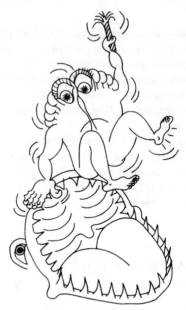

FLAT INSTEP: LACK OF SUPPORT!

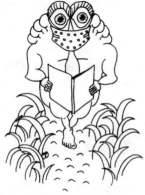

TENSE CERVICAL REFLEX: NOT TURNING TO OTHER POINTS OF VIEW!

Tense cervical reflex: Rigid thoughts and ideas due to insecurity. Narrow-mindedness limiting opportunity to enrich life's experiences. Reluctance to embrace the enormity and richness of life willingly.

Fallen arch: Collapsed support. The truth and foundation of life cease to exist.

FALLEN ARCH: DROWNING FROM LACK OF SUPPORT!

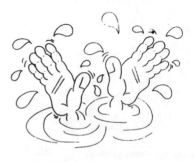

Rigid: Back against the wall. Unbending. Highly principled. Extremely insecure.

Rippled skin over bony reflex: Concerned and worried about support. Feeling overburdened and weighed down.

Sunken upper spinal reflex:
Perceived lack of emotional support. Giving in from carrying heavy emotional loads.

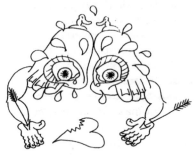

UNSUPPORTED UPPER BACK: NO EMOTIONAL SUPPORT!

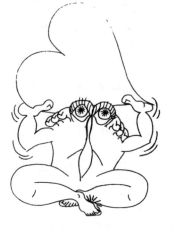

Swollen upper spinal reflex: Burdened with emotional responsibility.

OVERBURDENED UPPER BACK: WEIGHED DOWN WITH EMOTIONAL 'RESPONSIBILITY'!

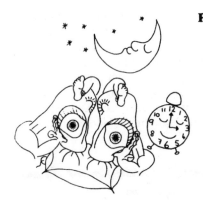

Protruding bone midway along bony ridge: Guilt regarding activities if above the waistline, or regarding relationships if below the waistline, or hidden resentment at the injustice of life. Disappointed that actions or communications have not met expectations.

THE GUILT BUMP!

Swollen around the ankle bone: Insecure due to reliance on materialism. Mistaken belief that money and possessions buy security leads to disillusionment and concern. As prisoners of possessions, movement becomes restricted and life limited to physical reality.

Smooth below inner ankle bone: No longer concerned about material possessions.

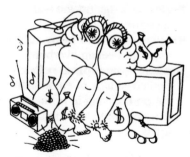

SWOLLEN INNER ANKLE: TRAPPED BY MATERIALISM!

Aching: Deep hurt and pain at all that is going on, particularly in the background.

Red along bony ridge: Anger at having the back put up, or at perceived lack of support, or from having to carry the load 'alone'.

THE EFFECT OF THE SUBCONSCIOUS MIND ON THE FLESHY INSTEP

Vibrant: In harmony with life.

Ridge of hard skin along the edge: Feeling divided. Difficulty in allowing the two-way exchange of life forces.

Swollen throat reflex: No time for the self. Too busy caring for others to the detriment of the self.

Swollen stomach reflex: Overwhelmed from having to take in and 'stomach' life's experiences.

Swelling midway: Guilty about feeling out of control or disappointed with achievements, considered inadequate since unrealistically high personal expectations are not met.

Swollen small intestine reflexes: (from the centre to the base of the ankle) Unable to sift through life's experiences. Difficulty in communicating or feeling entrapped within a relationship.

Money is an illusion and there are plenty more illusions were that came from

Swollen uterine reflex:
Unresolved issue related to femininity or reflecting an embryo six to eight weeks after conception. The latter is apparent on one foot only for single pregnancies, but is often visible on both feet if twins.

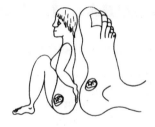

PREGNANT!

Broken blood vessels: Reflect inner trauma from emotional or physical abuse.

Red, puffy uterine reflex: Anger and frustration at infertility or inflamed that femininity is being taken advantage of. Frustrated communication.

Hard, white, flat uterine reflex: If lacking vibrancy and looks lifeless, indicates loss of life, particularly through miscarriage.

Broken blood vessels over reproductive reflexes: Possible sexual abuse or prejudice against females.

Swollen bladder reflex:
Frustration and anger particularly towards a partner. Extremely depressed. Pleasure and security threatened. In early pregnancy, the embryo reflex overlaps the bladder reflex. Towards the end of pregnancy, the baby's head, engaged in the pelvis, rebounds onto this part of the foot.

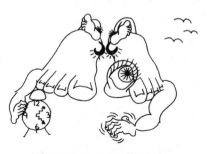

SWOLLEN BLADDER REFLEX

Swollen heel: Lacks security. Caught up in the materialism of the physical world. Reluctance to release past or fiercely protective of masculinity or femineity.

Reflexology footnote

✱ TO EASE BACKACHE AND NERVOUS STRAIN, PULL EACH PAIR OF TOES SIMULTANEOUSLY, STARTING WITH THE LITTLE TOES, BUT FIRST ENSURE THAT THE RECIPIENT IS LYING FLAT AND ABSOLUTELY STRAIGHT.

Cultural Influence on Feet

The cultural cultivation and sculpturing of feet.

The freedom and constraints of individual cultures leave their own particular mark and impression on the feet of its people.

Africans and Aborigines, adversely affected by a lack of recognition, share marked similarities. Insufficient support causes arches to drop, whilst the need for extra protection has resulted in thickened skin, with black marks displaying perceived abuse.

The bound feet of Chinese women reflect the constriction and bondage of females in a strictly male-dominated society. The toes were broken and bent before binding, to inhibit the amount of space for individual ideas and to discourage any participation or sharing of personal opinions. The smallness of their feet forbade a large impression from being made. Total subservience and bondage were inevitable, as outwardly manifested by the feet.

Particular types of thought-induced dis-eases inflict certain cultures due to mass belief systems and entrenched conditioning of society.

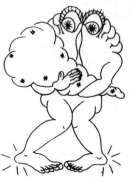

Cultural inhibitions

The greater the hardship, the greater the challenge!

CONCLUSION

In an age of doom and gloom, Reflexology and the Language of the Feet offer hope of fulfilment!

The increasing tendency to turn towards natural therapy arises from disillusionment at not finding solutions in the physical world for the total relief of bodily ailments. Drugs, alcohol, smoking and food can ease the physical symptoms of distress temporarily, but cannot dissipate the emotive causes, unless accompanied by a change of attitude. **The functioning of the mind and the functioning of the body cannot and should not be separated.**

A mind filled with constructive, encouraging messages enjoys a peaceful, more rewarding reality, but fears and anxieties buried deep in the recesses of the mind tend to defuse the initial enthusiasm to change.

This is where the feet step in!

Through the 'Language of the Feet', subconscious and unconscious thought patterns can be advantageously changed to relieve the monotony and frustration of life. Man's gift of free will can be used to release him from the shackles of self-imposed constraint.

'The Language of the Feet' is also a gift to mankind. Use this simple gift to change the direction of **your** life for the better, and find an inner peace and happiness that is beyond comprehension.

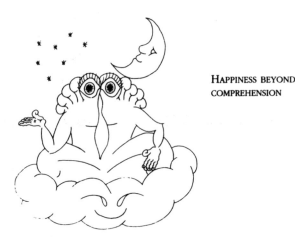

HAPPINESS BEYOND COMPREHENSION

APPENDIX I

THE ENERGIES OF THE LEFT AND RIGHT FEET

RIGHT FOOT	LEFT FOOT
Past.	Present/future.
Outgoing and giving.	Receptive and receiving.
The male energy of the Piscean Era.	The female energy of the Aquarian Age.
Positive. All past experiences can be used with positive effect.	Negative. Provides balance by questioning and testing the way.
Light exposed through past experiences.	Dark and mysterious, filled with the unknown.
Hollow and empty as the past is released.	Solid foundation for growth and development. The substance of life.
Main liver reflex. Stores past emotions.	Bulk of the stomach reflex. Anticipation of that which is to come.

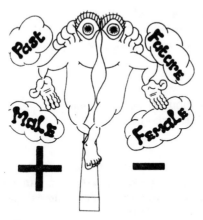

THE BALANCE BETWEEN THE RIGHT AND
LEFT FEET

Appendix II

Individual toes and their meanings

BIG TOE
Meaning: Thoughts, intellect, intuition and spirituality.
Connection: Nervous system and all toes.
Element: Ether.
Colour: Indigo/violet.
Relations: Thumb and toe necks.
Related reflexes: Head, brain, pituitary gland, pineal gland, thyroid gland, face, sensory organs, neck and throat.

SECOND TOE
Meaning: Loving thoughts regarding feelings, particularly of self-esteem and self-worth.
Connection: Respiratory system.
Element: Air.
Colour: Turquoise, blue, green.
Relations: Index finger and ball of foot.
Related reflexes: Shoulders, thyroid gland, thymus gland, chest, upper arm, upper spine, breast, solar plexus, heart, oesophagus, trachea, knee.

THIRD TOE
Meaning: Lively thoughts about activities and basic emotions.
Connections: Digestive system.
Element: Fire.
Colour: Yellow.
Relations: Third finger and upper instep.
Related reflexes: Solar plexus, heart, liver, pancreas, stomach, spleen, duodenum, transverse colon, adrenal glands, elbow, lower arm, hand, middle back.

FOURTH TOE
  Meaning: Pleasurable thoughts regarding communication and relationships.
  Connections: Circulatory, lymphatic and excretory systems.
  Element: Water.
  Colour: Orange.
  Relations: Ring finger and lower instep.
  Related reflexes: Small intestine, large colon, kidneys, ureter, uterus, Fallopian tubes, mid-spine, lower arms, lower legs.

LITTLE TOE
  Meaning: Expansive thoughts regarding family and security.
  Connections: Skeletal and muscular systems.
  Element: Earth.
  Colour: Red.
  Relations: Little finger and heel.
  Related reflexes: Pelvis, hip, feet, testes, prostate, ovaries, reproductive organs, lower spine, buttocks, bladder, rectum, anus.

Reflexology footnotes

* THE FOURTH TOE COMMONLY TURNS AND BENDS UNDER THE THIRD TOE, INDICATING EXTREME SHYNESS AND LACK OF CONFIDENCE ON THOSE WHO ARE AFRAID TO FACE THE WORLD OPENLY, SINCE THEIR OWN SPECIAL BRAND OF COMMUNICATION AND IDEAS SEEM TO BE SO DIFFERENT FROM ACCEPTED SOCIAL 'NORMS'.
* THE DEGREE OF BASHFULNESS IS DETERMINED BY THE AMOUNT OF MISALIGNMENT ON THE TOE.

Appendix III

Relationship between the big and second toes

RELATIONSHIP	BIG TOE	BOTH TOES	SECOND TOE
SUPPORTING	Intellectual, intuitive thoughts bolster self-esteem.	Intellect and self-esteem are inter-dependent.	Perceptions of personal capabilities encourage intellect.
SQUASHING	Intellectual pursuits leave little or no space to think of the self.	Inhibited intellect undermining self-worth.	Restricted space for personal thoughts.
KNOCKING	Thoughts of inadequacy belittle self-esteem and self-confidence.	Intellectual capabilities and self-perceptions continually conflict with one another.	Self-importance knocks need to think intelligently.
OVERLAPPING	Succumbs to other belief systems to the detriment of the self.	Not applicable.	Ego overshadows and dominates logical thought processes.
HIDING	Belief that the intellect is inadequate. Keeping ideas to the self.	Both toes behind the third toe. Intellectual and personal perceptions considered unworthy of scrutiny.	Holds back, or lacks confidence in self. Would rather not be noticed.
RESTING	Ideas propped by belief in self competency.	Intellect and personal perceptions dependent on one another.	Feelings for the self seek continual reassurance from the intellect.
HOLDING BACK	Keeps ideas to the self. Needs to step back to think.	Uncertainty regarding intellect and self-worth. Not wishing to participate or contribute ideas.	Reluctant to express the self openly. Needs space.
PROJECTING FORWARDS	Asserts own views above all else and seeks approval or acceptance.	Likes to be recognised for own ideas and to be identified with them.	Promoting self worth and trying to have feelings acknowledged.

RELATIONSHIP BETWEEN THE SECOND AND THIRD TOES

RELATIONSHIP	SECOND TOE	BOTH TOES	THIRD TOE
SUPPORTING	Thoughts of personal capabilities encourage participation.	Self-esteem and activities are inter-dependent on one another.	Self-esteem bolstered through thoughts of activities.
SQUASHING	Feelings about the self leave little space for personal achievement.	Little or no room for perceptions of the self or personal talents.	So busy pleasing others that there is little or no time for the self.
KNOCKING	Belief in personal inadequacy prevents certain ideas from being put into action.	Perceptions of the self and personal activity continually conflict with one another.	Knocks self-confidence and self-esteem, creating belief that incapable of undertaking certain activities.
OVERLAPPING	Active thoughts restricted by ego. Too full of self-importance to consider certain tasks.	Not applicable.	Actions undermine self-esteem and confidence, **or** prefers activities to remain anonymous.
HIDING	Unwilling to accept responsibility or be associated with actions.	Both hiding behind big or fourth toes. Activities and personal feelings kept out of sight.	Thoughts about activities kept secret. Conceals ideas to prevent exposure.
RESTING	Perceived personal talents encourage ideas to be put into action.	Thoughts of self-worth and activities rely on one another.	Self-esteem boosted through perceived capabilities.
HOLDING BACK	Reluctant to share own ideas for fear of exposing true feelings.	Hesitant about coming forward and doing things. Would rather stand back or do things in own way.	Unwilling to step in line or conform. Prefers to hold back before being committed.
PROJECTING FORWARDS	Seeking acknowledge-ment and recognition for personal concepts.	Projecting the self and promoting personal activities to gain attention.	Looking for approval and appreciation of personal pursuits.

RELATIONSHIP BETWEEN THIRD AND FOURTH TOES

RELATIONSHIP	THIRD TOE	BOTH TOES	FOURTH TOE
SUPPORTING	Active thoughts encourage communication and relationships.	Thoughts regarding actions and self-expression are inter-dependent upon one another.	Ability to communicate and good relationships enhance activities.
SQUASHING	Actions hamper open communication and restrict relationships.	Little or no time or space to communicate or put personal ideas into action.	Unable to communicate own ideas due to lack of space and an overactive mind.
KNOCKING to	Active thoughts deter personal relationships or open communication.	Thoughts of activity, communications and relationships collide with one another.	All talk and no action. Has own ideas of how communicate but is unable to do so.
OVERLAPPING	Do things without communicating thoughts and ideas. Secretive about activities.	Not applicable.	Full of ideas of how things should be done. The thinkers, not the doers!
HIDING	Keeps thoughts regarding activities to the self. Devious mind due to thoughts of insecurity.	Unable to expose ideas regarding activities and not prepared to communicate openly with others.	Communications and relationships kept in the background. Concealing expressions.
RESTING	Actions encourage communication and support relationships.	Actions, communications and relationships all inter-dependent.	Thoughts of communication and relationships encourage ideas being put into action.
HOLDING BACK	Standing in the background before committing thoughts to action.	Holding back thoughts regarding active communication and relationships.	Thoughts regarding communications and relationships taking a back seat.
PROJECTING FORWARDS	Assertively applying thoughts and putting them into action.	Promoting the self and seeking recognition for actions, communications and relationships.	Putting forward ideas regarding communication and relationships.

RELATIONSHIP BETWEEN FOURTH AND LITTLE TOES

RELATIONSHIP	FOURTH TOE	BOTH TOES	LITTLE TOE
SUPPORTING	Thoughts of communication and relationships encourage personal development.	Family communications and relationships depend upon one another.	Stable thoughts encourage open communication and relationships.
SQUASHING	Thoughts regarding communication and relationships leave no room for expansion.	Conflict between family beliefs and personal relationships.	Social conditioning inhibits communications and relationships.
KNOCKING	Interaction undermines the importance of self development or family relationships.	Rivalry between conditioned belief systems and personal thoughts of communication.	Perceptions of family or lack of security inhibit relationships and undermine self-confidence.
OVERLAPPING	Preoccupied with thoughts of communications and relationship, obliterating thoughts of mobility and hindering progress.	Not applicable.	If hooked, extremely insecure. Anchored to materialism through misconception that security is purely physical. Inhibited.
HIDING	Keeps ideas about communications and relationships in the dark.	Does not wish to expose ideas regarding social conditioning, communications and personal relationships.	Does not like to reveal true thoughts regarding security, mobility or family beliefs.
RESTING	Growth and development rely on communicative thoughts.	Stability, personal enhancement and communication all inter-dependent.	Perceptions of communication and relationships depend on reassurance and stability.
HOLDING BACK	Staying in the background and not sharing thoughts on communication and relationships.	Not wishing to expose ideas regarding stability and self-expression.	Reluctant to show insecurity and immobility with own ideas.
PROJECTING FORWARDS	Promoting personal ideas on communication and relationships.	Seeking acknowledgement for growth, development, and relationships.	Putting forward views or pushing ahead with ideas on personal growth and development.

AUTHOR'S FOOTNOTE

This unique book contains universal knowledge but the choice to utilise it is personal.

The 'quotable quotes' are not ascribed to any one person since they are common sayings that have been around, in one form or another, for centuries.

People and feet take on many forms, making it impossible to describe each and every characteristic in detail. The information provided in this book will, I hope, however, create a firm basis from which to grow and develop. The contents have been simplified for clarity and understanding and, although gaps are inevitable, combine the general knowledge available with your own intuition for insight that will amaze you!

If you would like to know more about the fascinating role of the feet in promoting and maintaining optimum physical and emotional health, you might like to read my introduction for absolute beginners *Reflexology: Headway Lifeguides* (Hodder & Stoughton, 1992) or my more comprehensive guide, *Reflexology: The Definitive Guide* (Hodder & Stoughton, 1995).

Finally, to all those special souls who bared their soles and souls to provide further information, my heartfelt thanks. May 'reading the feet' bring as much joy, and wonderment to you as it has to me!

Chris Stormer, 1995